T0362465

Inherited Bleeding Disorders

Editor

NATHAN T. CONNELL

HEMATOLOGY/ONCOLOGY CLINICS OF NORTH AMERICA

www.hemonc.theclinics.com

Consulting Editors
GEORGE P. CANELLOS
EDWARD J. BENZ Jr

December 2021 • Volume 35 • Number 6

ELSEVIER

1600 John F. Kennedy Boulevard ⚫ Suite 1800 ⚫ Philadelphia, Pennsylvania, 19103-2899

http://www.theclinics.com

HEMATOLOGY/ONCOLOGY CLINICS OF NORTH AMERICA Volume 35, Number 6
December 2021 ISSN 0889-8588, ISBN 13: 978-0-323-81337-2

Editor: Stacy Eastman
Developmental Editor: Ann Gielou M. Posedio

Hematology/Oncology Clinics (ISSN 0889-8588) is published bimonthly by Elsevier Inc., 360 Park Avenue South, New York, NY 10010-1710. Months of issue are February, April, June, August, October, and December. Business and Editorial Offices: 1600 John F. Kennedy Blvd., Ste. 1800, Philadelphia, PA 19103–2899. Customer Service Office: 3251 Riverport Lane, Maryland Heights, MO 63043. Periodicals postage paid at New York, NY and at additional mailing offices. Subscription prices are $456.00 per year (domestic individuals), $1150.00 per year (domestic institutions), $100.00 per year (domestic students/residents), $480.00 per year (Canadian individuals), $100.00 per year (Canadian students/residents), $1213.00 per year (Canadian institutions) $547.00 per year (international individuals), $1213.00 per year (international institutions), and $255.00 per year (international students/residents). International air speed delivery is included in all *Clinics* subscription prices. All prices are subject to change without notice. **POSTMASTER:** Send address changes to *Hematology/Oncology Clinics of North America*, Elsevier Health Sciences Division, Subscription Customer Service, 3251 Riverport Lane, Maryland Heights, MO 63043. Customer Service (orders, claims, online, change of address): Elsevier Health Sciences Division, Subscription **Customer Service, 3251 Riverport Lane, Maryland Heights, MO 63043. Tel: 1-800-654-2452 (U.S. and Canada); 314-447-8871 (outside U.S. and Canada). Fax: 314-447-8029. E-mail: journalscustomerservice-usa@elsevier.com (for print support)**; **journalsonlinesupport-usa@elsevier.com (for online support)**.

Reprints. For copies of 100 or more, of articles in this publication, please contact the Commercial Reprints Department, Elsevier Inc., 360 Park Avenue South, New York, New York 10010-1710; Tel.: 212-633-3874, Fax: 212-633-3820, E-mail: reprints@elsevier.com.

Hematology/Oncology Clinics of North America is covered in *MEDLINE/PubMed (Index Medicus), EMBASE/ Excerpta Medica, and BIOSIS.*

Contributors

CONSULTING EDITORS

GEORGE P. CANELLOS, MD
William Rosenberg Professor of Medicine, Department of Medical Oncology, Dana-Farber Cancer Institute, Boston, Massachusetts, USA

EDWARD J. BENZ Jr, MD
Professor, Pediatrics, Richard and Susan Smith Professor, Medicine, Professor, Genetics, Harvard Medical School, President and CEO Emeritus, Office of the President, Dana-Farber Cancer Institute, Boston, Massachusetts, USA

EDITOR

NATHAN T. CONNELL, MD, MPH
Assistant Professor of Medicine, Harvard Medical School, Associate Physician, Hematology Division, Department of Medicine, Clinical Chief of Hematology, Brigham and Women's Faulkner Hospital, Boston, Massachusetts, USA

AUTHORS

GLAIVY BATSULI, MD
Assistant Professor of Pediatrics, Aflac Cancer and Blood Disorders Center of Children's Healthcare of Atlanta, Department of Pediatrics, Emory University, Atlanta, Georgia, USA

ELISABETH M. BATTINELLI, MD, PhD
Assistant Professor of Medicine, Division of Hematology, Department of Medicine, Brigham and Women's Hospital, Harvard Medical School, Boston, Massachusetts, USA

MEGAN CHAIGNEAU, RN, MSc
Clinical Research Nurse and Nurse Coordinator, Inherited Bleeding Disorders Program of Southeastern Ontario, Department of Medicine, Queen's University, Kingston, Ontario, Canada

TRACEY A. CHEVES, BS, MT(ASCP)
Coagulation and Transfusion Medicine, Rhode Island Hospital, Warren Alpert Medical School of Brown University, Providence, Rhode Island, USA

NATHAN T. CONNELL, MD, MPH
Assistant Professor of Medicine, Harvard Medical School, Associate Physician, Hematology Division, Department of Medicine, Clinical Chief of Hematology, Brigham and Women's Faulkner Hospital, Boston, Massachusetts, USA

JEAN MARIE CONNORS, MD
Hematology Division, Brigham and Women's Hospital, Dana-Farber Cancer Institute, Harvard Medical School, Boston, Massachusetts, USA

SANDRA DEMARINIS, MS, MT(ASCP)
Coagulation and Transfusion Medicine, Rhode Island Hospital, Warren Alpert Medical School of Brown University, Providence, Rhode Island, USA

VERONICA H. FLOOD, MD
Professor, Department of Pediatrics, Medical College of Wisconsin and Versiti Blood Research Institute, Comprehensive Center for Bleeding Disorders, Milwaukee, Wisconsin, USA

PAULA D. JAMES, MD, FRCPC
Professor, Hematologist, Department of Medicine, Queen's University, Kingston, Ontario, Canada

PETER KOUIDES, MD
Clinical Professor of Medicine, Mary M. Gooley Hemophilia Center, Rochester Regional Health, Rochester, New York, USA

ARIELLE L. LANGER, MD, MPH
Division of Hematology, Brigham and Women's Hospital, Instructor in Medicine, Harvard Medical School, Boston, Massachusetts, USA

MAGDALENA DOROTA LEWANDOWSKA, MD
Hematologist, Indiana Hemophilia and Thrombosis Center, Indianapolis, Indiana, USA

MING YEONG LIM, MBBChir
Department of Internal Medicine, Division of Hematology and Hematologic Malignancies, University of Utah, Salt Lake City, Utah, USA

LYNN MALEC, MD, MSc
Assistant Professor of Medicine and Pediatrics, Versiti Blood Research Institute, Milwaukee, Wisconsin, USA

JORI E. MAY, MD
Division of Hematology/Oncology, The University of Alabama at Birmingham, Birmingham, Alabama, USA

RABIN NIROULA, MD
Assistant Professor, Warren Alpert Medical School of Brown University, Division of Hematology-Oncology, Rhode Island Hospital, The Miriam Hospital, Providence, Rhode Island, USA

MENAKA PAI, MSc, MD, FRCPC
McMaster University, Hamilton Health Sciences, Hamilton Regional Laboratory Medicine Program, Hamilton, Canada

ARI PELCOVITS, MD
Warren Alpert Medical School of Brown University, Division of Hematology-Oncology, Rhode Island Hospital, The Miriam Hospital, Providence, Rhode Island, USA

MARGARET V. RAGNI, MD, MPH
Medicine and Clinical Translational Research, Department of Medicine, Division Hematology/Oncology, University of Pittsburgh Medical Center, Hemophilia Center of Western Pennsylvania, Pittsburgh, Pennsylvania, USA

FRED SCHIFFMAN, MD
Sigal Family Professor of Humanistic Medicine, Vice Chair, Department of Medicine, Warren Alpert Medical School of Brown University, Division of Hematology-Oncology, Rhode Island Hospital, The Miriam Hospital, Providence, Rhode Island, USA

CRAIG D. SEAMAN, MD, MS
Department of Medicine, Division Hematology/Oncology, University of Pittsburgh Medical Center, Pittsburgh, Pennsylvania, USA

ROBERT F. SIDONIO, Jr, MD, MSc
Associate Professor of Pediatrics, Emory University, Atlanta, Georgia, USA

JOSEPH D. SWEENEY, MD, FACP, FRCPath
Coagulation and Transfusion Medicine, Rhode Island Hospital, Professor of Pathology and Laboratory Medicine, Warren Alpert Medical School of Brown University, Providence, Rhode Island, USA

FREDERICK D. TSAI, MD, PhD
Clinical Fellow in Hematology/Oncology, Division of Hematology, Department of Medicine, Brigham and Women's Hospital, Division of Hematologic Neoplasia, Department of Medical Oncology, Dana-Farber Cancer Institute, Harvard Medical School, Boston, Massachusetts, USA

ANGELA C. WEYAND, MD
Assistant Professor, Department of Pediatrics, University of Michigan Medical School, Ann Arbor, Michigan, USA

ALISA S. WOLBERG, PhD
UNC Department of Pathology and Laboratory Medicine, UNC Blood Research Center, Chapel Hill, North Carolina, USA

FREDERICO XAVIER, MD, MS
Department of Pediatrics, Division Hematology/Oncology, University of Pittsburgh Medical Center, Children's Hospital of Pittsburgh, Pittsburgh, Pennsylvania, USA

Contents

Approach to the patient with bleeding begins with a thorough bleeding, medical, and family history to determine the nature of bleeding and severity of bleeding symptoms. Use of a Bleeding Assessment Tool allows the clinician to obtain a comprehensive bleeding history and ultimately determine the individual bleeding score that reflects bleeding severity and is classifiable as either normal or abnormal. In the absence of significant findings within patient history or presenting symptoms clearly pointing to a specific bleeding pathology, an approach to laboratory investigation is presented that proceeds through first-line, second-line, and third-line testing.

In patients presenting with a suspect hereditary bleeding disorder a detailed bleeding history is first obtained. Testing proceeds in a tiered manner with platelet count, platelet morphology, platelet histogram, PFA-100, fibrinogen, prothrombin time, and activated partial thromboplastin time. More detailed testing includes von Willebrand factor, individual clotting factor assays, and platelet function testing. Next, testing for a dysfibrinogenemia, FXIII, or a fibrinolytic defect is considered. Hemostatic abnormality is not demonstrated in a fraction of patients. An approach to management in these patients, such as desmopressin or antifibrinolytic therapy, may be required and empiric use of blood component therapy is discouraged.

Bleeding disorders due to platelet dysfunction are a common hematologic complication affecting patients, and typically present with mucocutaneous bleeding or hemorrhage. An inherited platelet disorder should be suspected in individuals with a suggestive family history and no identified secondary causes of bleeding. Genetic defects have been described at all levels of platelet activation, including receptor binding, signaling, granule release, cytoskeletal remodeling, and platelet hematopoiesis. Management of these disorders is typically supportive, with an emphasis on awareness, patient education, and anticipatory guidance to prevent future episodes of bleeding.

Von Willebrand disease (VWD) is a common bleeding disorder, affecting male and female individuals equally, that often manifests in mucosal bleeding. VWD can be secondary to a quantitative (Type 1 and Type 3) or qualitative (Type 2) defects in Von Willebrand factor (VWF). Initial testing includes VWF antigen, as well as a platelet binding assay to differentiate between qualitative and quantitative defects. Further subtyping requires additional testing and is needed to ensure appropriate treatment. Desmopressin, antifibrinolytics, hormonal treatments for heavy menstrual bleeding, and VWF concentrates are commonly used in the treatment of VWD.

Acquired von Willebrand syndrome can occur in the setting of myeloproliferative neoplasms; plasma cell dyscrasias and other lymphoproliferative disorders; autoimmune conditions; and causes of increased shear forces, such as aortic stenosis or other structural heart disease and mechanical circulatory support. The depletion of von Willebrand factor, especially high-molecular-weight multimers, can lead to mucocutaneous bleeding and the formation of arteriovenous malformations, particularly in the gastrointestinal tract. Management focuses on correction of the underlying cause when possible, but may include intravenous immunoglobulins, von Willebrand factor concentrate, rituximab, or antiangiogenic therapy depending on the clinical context.

Remarkable changes are occurring in the diagnosis and management of individuals with hemophilia A. Genetic testing, including next-generation sequencing, enables family planning, carrier testing, and prenatal diagnosis. Musculoskeletal ultrasound examination facilitates the early detection of acute bleeds and joint disease in clinic, enabling more rapid bleed resolution and treatment planning. Novel therapies offer simpler weekly or monthly administration, some by subcutaneous injection, with better compliance and quality of life, as well as fewer bleeds. Gene therapy provides a 1-time phenotypic "cure" that is cost effective, but may be complicated by waning levels, vector immune responses, and hepatotoxicity.

Acquired hemophilia A is a potentially severe bleeding disorder caused by antibodies against the patient's own factor VIII. Acquired hemophilia A is rare. It is most commonly diagnosed in older individuals; about one-half of cases of acquired hemophilia are associated with underlying conditions, including autoimmune disease, cancer, and pregnancy. The diagnosis of acquired hemophilia A can be suspect with an isolated activated partial thromboplastin time elevation, and confirmed with demonstration of reduced factor VIII activity and the presence of a specific factor VIII inhibitor. Treatment of acquired hemophilia A involves control of bleeding, and eradication of the inhibitor.

factors play a critical role in the coagulation cascade. Incomplete bleeding evaluation or misinterpretation of laboratory studies can result in delayed diagnoses that ultimately affect patient outcomes. Bleeding manifestations can range from mild to severe, but the most common are mucocutaneous bleeding. The ideal treatment in RBD is dedicated single-factor concentrates that can be used for acute bleeding events, surgical management, and prophylaxis.

Fibrinogen plays a fundamental role in coagulation through its support for platelet aggregation and its conversion to fibrin. Fibrin stabilizes clots and serves as a scaffold and immune effector before being broken down by the fibrinolytic system. Given its importance, abnormalities in fibrin(ogen) and fibrinolysis result in a variety of disorders with hemorrhagic and thrombotic manifestations. This review summarizes (i) the basic elements of fibrin(-ogen) and its role in coagulation and the fibrinolytic system; (ii) the laboratory evaluation for fibrin(ogen) disorders, including the use of global fibrinolysis assays; and (iii) the management of congenital and acquired disorders of fibrinogen and fibrinolysis.

HEMATOLOGY/ONCOLOGY CLINICS OF NORTH AMERICA

SERIES OF RELATED INTEREST

Surgical Oncology Clinics of North America
https://www.surgonc.theclinics.com/

THE CLINICS ARE AVAILABLE ONLINE!
Access your subscription at:
www.theclinics.com

Preface

Inherited Bleeding Disorders

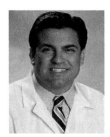

Nathan T. Connell, MD, MPH
Editor

Evaluation of the patient with a suspected bleeding disorder is both fascinating and frightening for the treating clinician given the broad differential diagnosis coupled with the potential for life-threatening symptoms. Across a diverse spectrum of causes, inherited bleeding disorders present a unique challenge due to the variability in clinical presentation, special requirements for diagnostic testing, and limited access to appropriate therapies for management. For many clinicians, the coagulation cascade is the epitome of a "black box" in their fund of knowledge; a complex set of biochemical reactions made even more confusing by the use of Roman numerals and arrows that cross one another in an attempt to describe the delicate homeostatic balance of hemostasis that is in reality much more complex than any single diagram could possibly convey.

The inherited bleeding disorders represent a complex and varied group of conditions centered on decreased ability for blood to generate or maintain thrombus. Even von Willebrand disease, the world's most common inherited bleeding disorder, is still considered a rare disease and is significantly underdiagnosed. The development of a structured approach to the history of patients with suspected bleeding disorders, such as the International Society on Thrombosis and Haemostasis Bleeding Assessment Tool, was intended to provide clinicians an opportunity to obtain a complete bleeding history, document the severity of symptoms to facilitate communication among clinicians, and standardize entry into clinical trials.

Coagulation testing is complex and expensive and requires significant specialized laboratory expertise. Preanalytic variables, such as the clinical condition of the patient, the manner in which the blood specimens are collected, and how they are transported to the laboratory, will all affect the quality and reliability of the results generated on the various testing platforms. For instance, a child who undergoes multiple attempts at venipuncture will likely have higher circulating von Willebrand factor levels than their usual baseline, potentially obscuring the diagnosis of hereditary von Willebrand

Hematol Oncol Clin N Am 35 (2021) xiii–xiv
https://doi.org/10.1016/j.hoc.2021.09.001
0889-8588/21/© 2021 Published by Elsevier Inc.

hemonc.theclinics.com

disease. Platelets are exquisitely sensitive to the handling and processing of the blood specimen and may partially activate during transport, leading to blunted responses on platelet aggregation and secretion assays.

In this issue of *Hematology/Oncology Clinics of North America*, I am grateful to my clinical and scientific colleagues for contributing their expertise to these articles on the current state of the science in the diagnosis and management of inherited bleeding disorders and closely related acquired bleeding conditions. Our collective hope for the bleeding disorder community is to make it easier for patients to obtain an accurate diagnosis and ensure access to appropriate treatment for the best possible quality of life.

Nathan T. Connell, MD, MPH
Brigham and Women's Hospital
Hematology Division, SR322
Boston, MA 02115, USA

E-mail address:
ntconnell@bwh.harvard.edu

Assessment of Bleeding

Approach to the Patient with Bleeding

Megan Chaigneau, RN, MSc, Paula D. James, MD, FRCPC*

KEYWORDS

- Bleeding score • Bleeding assessment tool (BAT) • Von Willebrand disease (VWD)
- Hemophilia • Platelet function disorder (PFD)

KEY POINTS

- Patient history includes bleeding, medical, and family history. Bleeding Assessment Tools allow the clinician to obtain a comprehensive and reproducible bleeding history that results in a bleeding score, classifiable as either normal or abnormal, with score magnitude reflecting bleeding severity.
- Clinical manifestations of bleeding disorders can be categorized into defects of primary hemostasis, defects of secondary hemostasis, and abnormalities of connective tissue/collagen. Each grouping has characteristic symptoms that may direct clinician to diagnostic category.
- Significant findings within the individual patient history or presenting symptoms may point to a specific pathology that can be confirmed with laboratory investigation.
- In the absence of significant findings, a sequential method of laboratory investigation is presented, starting with first-line screening tests, second-line testing to identify the most common bleeding disorders (VWD and PFD), and finally third-line testing for rarer disorders.
- Despite extensive testing and a significant bleeding pathology, some patients will remain undiagnosed and can be categorized as having bleeding of unknown cause.

INTRODUCTION

The approach to a patient with bleeding begins with a thorough review of the personal bleeding and medical history, as well as family history. The use of bleeding assessment tools (BATs) facilitates the clinician in obtaining a complete and accurate assessment of bleeding symptoms while allowing for objective documentation of those that are outside of the normal range. Physical examination aids in corroborating symptoms and should be guided by the patient's bleeding history. Laboratory investigation is also guided by both bleeding and family history; however, von Willebrand disease (VWD)

Department of Medicine, Queen's University, Room 2015, Etherington Hall, 94 Stuart Street, Kingston, Ontario K7L 3N6, Canada
* Corresponding author.
E-mail address: jamesp@queensu.ca

Hematol Oncol Clin N Am 35 (2021) 1039–1049
https://doi.org/10.1016/j.hoc.2021.07.001
0889-8588/21/© 2021 Elsevier Inc. All rights reserved.

hemonc.theclinics.com

should be considered within the broad differential, as it is the most common and best characterized of the primary hemostatic disorders. Clinical management is highly individualized, focusing on the specific bleeding disorder and clinical manifestations experienced by the patient. Finally, despite extensive testing and clinical evidence of abnormal bleeding, there will remain many patients who are not categorizable within a specific diagnosis and could be considered to have bleeding of unknown cause (BUC).

DISCUSSION
Patient History: Bleeding History (Use of Bleeding Assessment Tools), Medical and Family History

The first step in the assessment of the patient with bleeding is evaluation of the patient's history, including bleeding, medical, and family history. A thorough bleeding history requires documentation of all aspects of abnormal bleeding symptoms, including frequency, onset, severity, need for medical intervention, associated bleeding complications, and outcome of past hemostatic challenges. Bleeding histories are inherently subjective, and the quality of the obtained history can be influenced by factors related to the patient, such as education level, but also by the clinician's individual interpretation of reported symptoms.[1,2] Much work to standardize bleeding histories has been undertaken over the years in an effort to reduce subjectivity and improve their overall quality, reproducibility, and diagnostic utility. A BAT generally consists of a standardized bleeding questionnaire and a well-defined interpretation grid used to determine bleeding score. Many BATs have been published, including the "Vicenza Bleeding Questionnaire,"[3] Molecular and Clinical Markers for the Diagnosis and Management of Type 1 von Willebrand disease (MCDM-1 VWD),[4] Condensed MCDM-1 VWD,[5] and the Pediatric Bleeding Questionnaire.[6] In 2010, much of this work was consolidated with the publication of the International Society of Thrombosis and Haemostasis BAT (ISTH-BAT), which targets both adult and pediatric patients who are being evaluated for a bleeding disorder for the first time.[7]

The ISTH-BAT can be used by any physician or other trained health-professional without the need for specific hematology expertise. The user is guided through 14 sections outlined in **Box 1**, each addressing a specific bleeding domain with the final domain covering childhood-specific hemorrhagic symptoms. Detailed subquestions within the questionnaire cover key aspects such as frequency and duration of symptoms, age of onset, and level of medical intervention required. The information gathered allows the clinician to determine symptom significance and assign a representative score via the scoring key. For each category, the patient receives a score ranging from 0 to 4 based on the most severe instance of each symptom, with the overall sum representing the final bleeding score. The normal range has been determined as 0 to 3 for men, 0 to 5 for women, and 0 to 2 for both male and female children.[8] The full ISTH-BAT questionnaire and scoring key can be found online at https://www.isth.org/page/reference_tools.

In general, BATs serve first as a screening tool for individuals being investigated for a suspected bleeding disorder, and second, as a standardized way of describing disease characteristics, and assessing overall bleeding severity.[1] They have clinical utility in any setting where bleeding is of concern and a comprehensive bleeding history needs to be taken. Recommendations for their use as a screening tool in different settings are described in this article and are aligned with the recently published guidelines on the diagnosis of VWD.[9] Within a primary care setting, there is a strong indication for

Box 1
Bleeding domains assessed within International Society of Thrombosis and Haemostasis Bleeding Assessment Tool (ISTH-BAT)

1. Epistaxis
2. Cutaneous bleeding
3. Bleeding from minor wounds
4. Oral cavity
5. Gastrointestinal bleeding
6. Hematuria
7. Tooth extraction
8. Surgery
9. Menorrhagia
10. Postpartum hemorrhage
11. Muscle hematoma
12. Hemarthrosis
13. Central nervous system bleeding
14. Other bleeding: umbilical stump bleeding, cephalohematoma, cheek hematoma caused by sucking during breast/bottle feeding, conjunctival hemorrhage, or excessive bleeding following circumcision or venipuncture

the use of a validated BAT to aid the clinician in determining which patients warrant a referral for more focused investigation.[10,11] Within a hematology referral population for abnormal bleeding or screening tests, there remains a strong indication for the use of BATs. However, for this setting in which the probability of having a bleeding disorder is higher than in a general primary care population, the bleeding score alone should not be the sole determination of whether further testing is required. In this population, the BAT should be used in conjunction with specific laboratory testing at the discretion of the hematologist to complete the initial diagnostic approach. Finally, for patients with a high probability of having an inherited bleeding disorder (eg, affected first-degree relative), a BAT may still be used to gather the bleeding history but referral to hematology and further laboratory testing should be performed regardless of bleeding score.

One limitation of the ISTH-BAT is the need for expert-administration by a physician or other trained health care personnel. This issue was addressed with the creation of the self-administered BAT (Self-BAT) via a multiphase study that modified the ISTH-BAT for self-administration.[12] The Self-BAT demonstrated bleeding scores comparable to the ISTH-BAT,[12] has identical normal ranges,[8] and has been validated for use as a screening tool in a hematology clinic,[12] in patients with suspected congenital platelet defects,[13] and modified for the pediatric population.[14] An electronic version of the Self-BAT can be accessed online at www.letstalkperiod.ca/self-bat with users receiving their bleeding score and a printable pdf of their results on completion of the test.[15]

Expanded use of BATs has been proposed for resource-limited settings where there are significant challenges in accessing laboratory testing. Many low-income and middle-income countries have very limited access to specialized hemostatic testing, with the available testing of varying quality, poorly accessible, and at significant cost to the patient.[16,17] Regional use of BATs in these settings has been proposed as a cost-effective way to standardize evaluation of clinically significant bleeding at the primary care level, and determine for which individuals laboratory testing is justified.[16,17] This will require future research to develop and validate BAT translations that appropriately account for the cultural, religious, geographic, and socioeconomic factors specific to each region or country.

In addition to bleeding history, medical and family history also must be discussed. Evaluation of medical history includes investigation into comorbidities such as renal disease, liver disease, and autoimmune disease, as well as a detailed review of medications, with particular attention to the use of aspirin (ASA), nonsteroidal anti-inflammatory drugs (NSAIDs), anticoagulants, clopidogrel, and herbal supplements. Evaluation of family history requires discussion of first-degree relatives, looking for the presence of hemostatic disorders or other undiagnosed but symptomatic family members. Significant information within the medical or family history may clearly point to a specific bleeding pathogenesis, whether acquired or inherited.

Physical Examination

Physical examination is somewhat limited, as many symptoms are transient and may not be present at the time of a patient's appointment. It may include the following:

- Inspection of the skin for signs of petechiae, ecchymoses, telangiectasia, and abnormal scarring
- Signs of anemia
- Joint examination if positive history for hemarthrosis
- Assessment of facial or skeletal anomalies
- Assessment of joint hypermobility using the Beighton Scale[18]
- Assessment for cardiac murmurs, lymphadenopathy, splenomegaly, hepatomegaly, thyroid goiter, evidence of cirrhosis

Clinical Manifestations

The typical clinical manifestations of bleeding disorders can be roughly categorized into defects of primary hemostasis, defects of secondary hemostasis, and abnormalities of connective tissue/collagen. The usual pattern of clinical symptoms for each category are summarized within the sections that follow. Presenting symptoms may be influenced by comorbidities and/or medications, with some symptoms only becoming apparent after a hemostatic challenge, such as menses, surgery, or trauma. If a patient presents with a new onset of bleeding symptoms and has a negative past personal and family history, consideration should be made for an acquired bleeding disorder, which can affect any of the components of hemostasis.

Defects of primary hemostasis

The 2 most common defects of primary hemostasis are VWD and platelet function disorder (PFDs). Both will present with characteristic mucocutaneous bleeding symptoms including ecchymoses, epistaxis, heavy menstrual bleeding, and excessive bleeding after minor wounds, dental extractions, surgery, childbirth, and bleeding from the oral cavity and gastrointestinal (GI) tract. When faced with a hemostatic challenge, bleeding is immediate. In contrast, musculoskeletal bleeding and other severe bleeding symptoms (central nervous system or GI tract) are rare and typically observed only in severe forms of VWD or PFD.[19]

Defects of secondary hemostasis

Defects of secondary hemostasis result from deficiencies or defects in coagulation factors. The most well-known disorders are Hemophilia A (HA) and Hemophilia B

(HB), which result from deficiencies in Factor VIII (FVIII) and Factor IX (FIX), respectively; however, other coagulation factors can be deficient. Coagulation factor deficiency typically manifests as deep tissue bleeding, including large palpable ecchymoses, deep soft tissue hematomas, intramuscular hematomas, and musculoskeletal bleeding such as hemarthrosis. Mild deficiencies may only present after hemostatic challenges with delayed postsurgical bleeding complications. Mucocutaneous bleeding symptoms like epistaxis may still be observed, but any presence of deep tissue bleeding or delayed bleeding should guide the clinician toward a defect of secondary hemostasis.

Abnormalities of connective tissue/collagen

Ehlers Danlos syndrome comprises a heterogeneous group of connective tissue disorders with clinical symptoms that reflect vascular fragility. Easy or spontaneous bruising is often the presenting complaint and recurs in the same areas, causing a characteristic discoloration of the skin from hemosiderin deposition.[20] A wide range of other bleeding symptoms can be observed, such as subcutaneous hematomas, oral mucosal bleeding, and heavy menstrual bleeding, along with more severe internal bleeding as a result of arterial rupture. Bleeding complications with hemostatic challenge are immediate.[21] Other nonbleeding clinical manifestations include joint hypermobility, skin hyperextensibility, delayed wound healing, atrophic scarring, and generalized connective tissue fragility.[20,21]

Investigation

A strategy for laboratory investigation of the patient with bleeding is outlined in **Table 1**. The approach begins with a series of screening tests, along with additional investigations to identify common causes and consequences of bleeding disorders. If family history clearly points to a certain disorder, appropriate investigations for that specific disorder should be included in the first-line testing. Any abnormalities in screening tests should be pursued, with detailed interpretation of screening tests outlined in **Table 2**. Otherwise, progression to second-line testing aims to identify VWD and PFD, as these 2 diagnoses represent the most commonly diagnosed bleeding disorders. If no abnormality has been discovered at this point, third-line testing of factor assays, fibrinolysis, and thrombin generation completes the available diagnostic workup, albeit with low diagnostic yield.[22] Patients with significant bleeding histories but unremarkable laboratory testing, may be classified as having BUC.[23]

Differential Diagnosis

The differential diagnosis for patients presenting with bleeding symptoms is broad, but information gathered via patient history and laboratory investigation may clearly point to specific disorders. **Fig. 1** summarizes both the overall diagnostic approach to the patient with bleeding and lists the disorders to be considered within the differential.

Treatment

Treatment options are highly dependent on the underlying bleeding disorder, disease severity, presenting symptoms, and anticipated hemostatic challenges. It can be roughly categorized into 4 areas:

1. General bleeding education:
   a. Importance of localized measures to control bleeding, including direct pressure, compression, and use of ice/cold pack.
   b. Instructions to avoid medications that exacerbate bleeding tendencies, such as ASA, NSAIDs, and certain alternative medications.

Table 1
Suggested approach to laboratory investigation

Type of Testing	Additional Details
First line	
• If patient history clearly indicates a particular disorder, appropriate investigations should be performed at first-line testing; for example, if family history of HB, FIX level should be included	
Screening tests: • CBC with differential, PT, aPTT, TT, fibrinogen	• CBC with differential assesses the platelet count and allows for morphologic assessment of all the cell lines • See **Table 2** for detailed interpretation of PT, aPTT, TT and fibrinogen
• Ferritin	• To identify iron deficiency, a common consequence of bleeding disorders
• Renal and liver function tests, thyroid stimulating hormone (TSH)	• When clinically indicated, may identify common, easily diagnosable causes of acquired bleeding disorders
• Bleeding time (BT) • Platelet function analyzer 100 (PFA-100)	• BT is an in vivo hemostasis test of questionable utility, but may be useful in settings where second-line and third-line testing is not available.[24] • PFA-100 measures platelet function under conditions of high shear. It is abnormal in patients with severe PFD but also lacks sensitivity in persons with mild bleeding.[24,25]
Second line	
• In presence of normal screening tests, second-line testing aims to identify the 2 most common causes of mild to moderate bleeding disorders, VWD and PFD	

• VWD Testing:
   ○ VWF:Ag
   ○ VWF:GPIbM
   ○ FVIII
• Platelet function testing (PFT)
	• VWD testing includes a measure of the quantity of VWF protein in the plasma (VWF:Ag), a measure of the platelet-dependent VWF activity (VWF:GPIbM), and an FVIII assay, as VWF functions is the carrier protein for FVIII in the plasma. See consensus guidelines for the diagnostic criteria of each VWD subtype.[9]
	• PFT includes light transmission aggregometry and electron microscopy. Tests are time-consuming and subject to significant preanalytical and analytical variables. See consensus guidelines for abnormalities that suggest specific diagnoses.[26]

Third line	
• Can be considered in presence of abnormal screening tests or in cases of severe bleeding symptoms with unremarkable first-line and second-line testing	
• Factor assays (ex. II, V, VII, IX, XI, XIII) • Mixing studies • Inhibitor assays • Urea clot stability or euglobulin clot lysis time	• Factor assays for FIX and FVIII should be considered, as their deficiencies comprise the 2 most common hemophilias (unless FVIII was assessed with VWF testing in second line).[27]

(continued on next page)

Table 1 (continued)	
Type of Testing	Additional Details
• α_2-Antiplasmin level and plasminogen activator inhibitor activity • Reptilase time	Other factor deficiencies are rare but are more common in certain populations (FXI deficiency in the Ashkenazi Jewish population) and consanguineous families.[27,28]

Abbreviations: aPTT, activated partial thromboplastin time; FVIII, factor VIII; FXI, factor XI; HB, hemophilia B; PFD, platelet function disorder; PT, prothrombin time; TT, thrombin time; VWD, von Willebrand disease; VWF, von Willebrand factor

Adapted from Rydz N, James PD. Why is my patient bleeding or bruising? *Hematology/Oncology Clinics.* 2012;26(2):321-344; *with permission.*

   c. Encouragement to promptly seek medical attention when faced with any significant bleeding symptoms.

2. Assessment/treatment for common consequences of bleeding disorders:
   a. Screening for Hepatitis B, Hepatitis C, and human immunodeficiency virus if patient received either blood products or plasma-derived clotting factor concentrates before 1985, followed by vaccinations for Hepatitis A and Hepatitis B.[29]
   b. Gynecologic evaluation for women with heavy menstrual bleeding.[30] If available, referral should be made to a women and bleeding disorders clinic.
   c. Monitoring for iron deficiency and iron deficiency anemia with subsequent treatment when applicable.

3. Indirect therapies:

Table 2
Detailed interpretation of abnormal screening coagulation tests

PT	aPTT	TT	Fibrinogen	Interpretation
N	N	N	N	Normal profile, can be seen with mild factor deficiencies, mild VWD, PFD, FXIII deficiency, PAI-1 deficiency, α_2-Antiplasmin deficiency, and connective tissue disorders
↑	N	N	N	FVII deficiency, warfarin therapy, early liver failure, early DIC (disseminated intravascular coagulation)
N	↑	N	N	Deficiencies of FVIII, I, XI, XII, VWD if FVIII is significantly decreased
↑	↑	N	N	Deficiencies of FII, FV, FX; supratherapeutic warfarin
↑	↑	↑	↓	Dysfibrinogenemia or afibrinogenemia; late DIC or liver failure
↑	↑	↑	N	Large amounts of heparin (reptilase time is normal)
N	N	↑	↓	Mild cases of dysfibrinogenemia or hypofibrinogenemia
N	↑	↑	N	Heparin (reptilase time is normal)

Abbreviations: ↑, increased; ↓, decreased; aPTT, activated partial thromboplastin time; F, factor; HB, hemophilia B; N, normal; PAI-1, plasminogen activator inhibitor 1; PFD, platelet function disorder; PT, prothrombin time; TT, thrombin time; VWD, von Willebrand disease.

From Rydz N, James PD. Why is my patient bleeding or bruising? *Hematology/Oncology Clinics.* 2012;26(2):321-344; *with permission.*

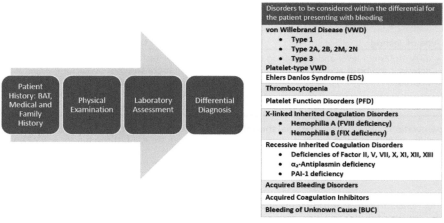

Fig. 1. Overall approach to the patient with bleeding.

   a. Fibrinolytic inhibitors, such as tranexamic acid, can be helpful treatment for a wide range of bleeding disorders, either as a primary treatment or adjunct to other therapy depending on the specific clinical situation.[29–32]

   b. Hormonal treatment with the oral contraceptive pill, use of an intrauterine device, and endometrial ablation can all be effective for the treatment of heavy menstrual bleeding in patients with bleeding disorders. Refer to consensus document on the management of abnormal gynecologic and obstetric bleeding in women with bleeding disorders.[30]

   c. Desmopressin therapy stimulates secretion of VWF from endothelial cells and may provide adequate hemostatic coverage for most invasive procedures. A test dose followed by serial measurements is necessary, as individual responsiveness can vary greatly.[33] The best defined indications for use of desmopressin in bleeding disorders are for VWD and HA, in mild to moderate disease,[34–36] but it has also been studied in other disorders.[37,38]

4. Direct/replacement therapies:

   a. Includes products that directly increase the plasma levels of the specific hemostatic defect. Clinicians should refer to the appropriate disease-specific guidelines for further information, such as those for VWD[39] and hemophilia.[40]

   b. In the case of refractory bleeding or in the presence of an inhibitor, bypassing agents may be considered (eg, recombinant Factor VIIa and Factor VIII inhibitor bypass activity).

SUMMARY

The overall approach to the patient with bleeding begins with a thorough history covering bleeding, medical, and family history, but requires confirmation and further direction via detailed laboratory investigation. Clinical manifestations will depend on the underlying bleeding pathology with significant overlap occurring among the various bleeding disorders, particularly those of mild severity characterized by mucocutaneous symptoms. The initial differential diagnosis is wide-ranging, but information gathered via history and results from laboratory investigations may help narrow down the possibilities and point to a specific disorder or category of disorders. Major challenges are the broad differential and highly specialized laboratory investigations required. Future directions for research include optimizing treatment strategies and further work to predict risk of future bleeding.

CLINICS CARE POINTS

- Several BATs have been validated and may be used in a variety of settings. For example, a condensed tool could be used in time-restricted settings or a self-administered tool in settings where access to a health care professional is limited.

- Pediatric patients may not have experienced hemostatic challenges and depending on age, may lack an established pattern of bleeding behaviors. There is also significant overlap between normal childhood issues and symptoms of mild bleeding disorders (eg, epistaxis and bruising). Differentiating between pathologic and normal bleeding is even more difficult in this population, and a negative bleeding history does not rule out bleeding diathesis.

- Presence of a bleeding disorder within a first-degree relative is a strong indication for specific laboratory investigation regardless of bleeding history.

- Laboratory findings should be interpreted with caution, as they are highly influenced by quality of the laboratory and other preanalytical variables. For example, VWD testing is affected by several environmental factors, including physiologic stressors and hormones, thus baseline testing should be avoided in stressed, ill, or pregnant patients when possible.

- The importance of women's symptoms, such as heavy menstrual bleeding and postpartum bleeding, should not be overlooked, as they play a significant role in achieving diagnosis.

- Patients ultimately classified as BUC should not be dismissed from hematology care and may need treatment for moderate and severe symptoms or in the event of high-risk hemostatic challenges.

DISCLOSURE

P. James has research funding from Bayer.

REFERENCES

1. Rydz N, James PD. The evolution and value of bleeding assessment tools. J Thromb Haemost 2012;10(11):2223–9.
2. Mauer AC, Khazanov NA, Levenkova N, et al. Impact of sex, age, race, ethnicity and aspirin use on bleeding symptoms in healthy adults. J Thromb Haemost 2011;9(1):100–8.
3. Rodeghiero F, Castaman G, Tosetto A, et al. The discriminant power of bleeding history for the diagnosis of type 1 von Willebrand disease: an international, multi-center study. J Thromb Haemost 2005;3(12):2619–26.
4. Tosetto A, Rodeghiero F, Castaman G, et al. A quantitative analysis of bleeding symptoms in type 1 von Willebrand disease: results from a multicenter European study (MCMDM-1 VWD). J Thromb Haemost 2006;4(4):766–73.
5. Bowman M, Mundell G, Grabell J, et al. Generation and validation of the condensed MCMDM-1VWD bleeding questionnaire for von Willebrand disease. J Thromb Haemost 2008;6(12):2062–6.
6. Bowman M, Riddel J, Rand M, et al. Evaluation of the diagnostic utility for von Willebrand disease of a pediatric bleeding questionnaire. J Thromb Haemost 2009; 7(8):1418–21.
7. Rodeghiero F, Tosetto A, Abshire T, et al. ISTH/SSC bleeding assessment tool: a standardized questionnaire and a proposal for a new bleeding score for inherited bleeding disorders. J Thromb Haemost 2010;8(9):2063–5.

8. Elbatarny M, Mollah S, Grabell J, et al. Normal range of bleeding scores for the ISTH-BAT: adult and pediatric data from the merging project. Haemophilia. 2014; 20(6):831–5.

9. James PD, Connell NT, Ameer B, et al. ASH ISTH NHF WFH 2021 guidelines on the diagnosis of von Willebrand disease. Blood Adv 2021;5(1):280–300.

10. Adler M, Kaufmann J, Alberio L, et al. Diagnostic utility of the ISTH bleeding assessment tool in patients with suspected platelet function disorders. J Thromb Haemost 2019;17(7):1104–12.

11. Gresele P, Orsini S, Noris P, et al. Validation of the ISTH/SSC bleeding assessment tool for inherited platelet disorders: a communication from the Platelet Physiology SSC. J Thromb Haemost 2020;18(3):732–9.

12. Deforest M, Grabell J, Albert S, et al. Generation and optimization of the self-administered bleeding assessment tool and its validation as a screening test for von Willebrand disease. Haemophilia. 2015;21(5):e384–8.

13. Punt MC, Blaauwgeers MW, Timmer MA, et al. Reliability and feasibility of the self-administered ISTH-bleeding assessment tool. TH Open 2019;3(4):e350.

14. Casey LJ, Tuttle A, Grabell J, et al. Generation and optimization of the self-administered pediatric bleeding questionnaire and its validation as a screening tool for von Willebrand disease. Pediatr Blood Cancer 2017;64(10):e26588.

15. Reynen E, Grabell J, Ellis A, et al. Let's talk period! Preliminary results of an online bleeding awareness knowledge translation project and bleeding assessment tool promoted on social media. Haemophilia. 2017;23(4):e282–6.

16. Rashid A, Moiz B, Karim F, et al. Use of ISTH bleeding assessment tool to predict inherited platelet dysfunction in resource constrained settings. Scand J Clin Lab Invest 2016;76(5):373–8.

17. Srivastava A. Diagnosis of haemophilia and other inherited bleeding disorders-is a new paradigm needed? Haemophilia 2021;27(Suppl 3):14–20.

18. Beighton P, Solomon L, Soskolne C. Articular mobility in an African population. Ann Rheum Dis 1973;32(5):413.

19. Mishra P, Naithani R, Dolai T, et al. Intracranial haemorrhage in patients with congenital haemostatic defects. Haemophilia 2008;14(5):952–5.

20. Paepe AD, Malfait F. Bleeding and bruising in patients with Ehlers–Danlos syndrome and other collagen vascular disorders. Br J Haematol 2004;127(5): 491–500.

21. Malfait F, De Paepe A. Bleeding in the heritable connective tissue disorders: mechanisms, diagnosis and treatment. Blood Rev 2009;23(5):191–7.

22. Rydz N, James PD. Why is my patient bleeding or bruising? Hematol Oncol Clin 2012;26(2):321–44.

23. Quiroga T, Goycoolea M, Panes O, et al. High prevalence of bleeders of unknown cause among patients with inherited mucocutaneous bleeding. A prospective study of 280 patients and 299 controls. Haematologica 2007;92(3):357–65.

24. Quiroga T, Goycoolea M, Munoz B, et al. Template bleeding time and PFA-100® have low sensitivity to screen patients with hereditary mucocutaneous hemorrhages: comparative study in 148 patients. J Thromb Haemost 2004;2(6):892–8.

25. Podda G, Bucciarelli P, Lussana F, et al. Usefulness of PFA-100® testing in the diagnostic screening of patients with suspected abnormalities of hemostasis: comparison with the bleeding time. J Thromb Haemost 2007;5(12):2393–8.

26. Hayward CP, Moffat KA, Raby A, et al. Development of North American consensus guidelines for medical laboratories that perform and interpret platelet function testing using light transmission aggregometry. Am J Clin Pathol 2010; 134(6):955–63.

27. Mannucci PM, Tuddenham EG. The hemophilias—from royal genes to gene therapy. N Engl J Med 2001;344(23):1773–9.
28. Asakai R, Chung DW, Davie EW, et al. Factor XI deficiency in Ashkenazi Jews in Israel. N Engl J Med 1991;325(3):153–8.
29. Nichols WL, Rick ME, Ortel TL, et al. Clinical and laboratory diagnosis of von Willebrand disease: a synopsis of the 2008 NHLBI/NIH guidelines. Am J Hematol 2009;84(6):366–70.
30. James AH, Kouides PA, Abdul-Kadir R, et al. Von Willebrand disease and other bleeding disorders in women: consensus on diagnosis and management from an international expert panel. Am J Obstet Gynecol 2009;201(1):12.e1–18.
31. Bonomi B. Guidelines on replacement therapy for haemophilia and inherited coagulation disorders in Italy. Haemophilia. 2000;6(1):1–10.
32. Geerts WH, Bergqvist D, Pineo GF, et al. Prevention of venous thromboembolism: American College of Chest Physicians evidence-based clinical practice guidelines. Chest. 2008;133(6):381S–453S.
33. Connell NT, James PD, Brignardello-Petersen R, et al. von Willebrand disease: proposing definitions for future research. Blood Adv 2021;5(2):565–9.
34. Castaman G, Lethagen S, Federici AB, et al. Response to desmopressin is influenced by the genotype and phenotype in type 1 von Willebrand disease (VWD): results from the European Study MCMDM-1VWD. Blood The J Am Soc Hematol 2008;111(7):3531–9.
35. Federici A. The use of desmopressin in von Willebrand disease: the experience of the first 30 years (1977–2007). Haemophilia 2008;14:5–14.
36. Franchini M, Zaffanello M, Lippi G. The use of desmopressin in mild hemophilia A. Blood Coagul Fibrinolysis 2010;21(7):615–9.
37. Bolton-Maggs PH, Chalmers EA, Collins PW, et al. A review of inherited platelet disorders with guidelines for their management on behalf of the UKHCDO. Br J Haematol 2006;135(5):603–33.
38. Franchini M, Manzato F, Salvagno GL, et al. The use of desmopressin in congenital factor XI deficiency: a systematic review. Ann Hematol 2009;88(10):931–5.
39. Connell NT, Flood VH, Brignardello-Petersen R, et al. ASH ISTH NHF WFH 2021 guidelines on the management of von Willebrand disease. Blood Adv 2021;5(1):301–25.
40. Srivastava A, Santagostino E, Dougall A, et al. WFH guidelines for the management of hemophilia. Haemophilia. 2020;26:1–158.

Laboratory Methods in the Assessment of Hereditary Hemostatic Disorders

Tracey A. Cheves, BS, MT(ASCP), Sandra DeMarinis, MS, MT(ASCP), Joseph D. Sweeney, MD, FRCPath*

KEYWORDS

- Hereditary bleeding disorders • Laboratory investigation • Hemostasis
- Fibrinolytic system

KEY POINTS

- The most important part of the investigation of a suspected hereditary bleeding disorder is the detailed clinical history.
- The investigation should start with basic screening tests, such as the platelet count, platelet morphology, platelet histogram, PFA-100, fibrinogen, PT, and aPTT.
- The next level of investigation is assessment of von Willebrand factor using antigenic and functional assays, aggregometry to detect a functional platelet defect, and individual clotting factor assays as indicated by the PT and aPTT.
- If the above testing does not reveal an abnormality, testing for a dysfibrinogenemia, assay of FXIII, or testing for a fibrinolytic disorder may be considered.

A HISTORY OF TESTING FOR INHERITED BLEEDING DISORDERS

By the beginning of the twentieth century, the then classical theory of blood coagulation held that tissue juice (thrombokinase, thromboplastin) complexed with prothrombin, converted prothrombin into thrombin, which, in the presence of calcium, converted fibrinogen to fibrin, resulting in the clotting of blood.[1–4] Hemophilia had long been known as a severe bleeding disorder, but the cause was unknown, possibly a deficiency of prothrombin. In 1913, Lee and White[5] described their whole blood clotting time in which blood was collected by venipuncture, placed into two glass tubes, and allowed to clot. They also discussed clot retraction, noting that patients with hemophilia had a prolonged clotting time (>50 minutes) but essentially normal clot retraction. Around the same time (1910), Duke[6] described his ear lobe bleeding time in the

Coagulation and Transfusion Medicine, Rhode Island Hospital and Warren Alpert School of Medicine at Brown University, 593 Eddy Street, Providence, RI 02903, USA
* Corresponding author. Transfusion Medicine, Rhode Island Hospital, 593 Eddy Street, Providence, RI 02903.
E-mail address: jsweeney@lifespan.org

Hematol Oncol Clin N Am 35 (2021) 1051–1068
https://doi.org/10.1016/j.hoc.2021.07.002
0889-8588/21/© 2021 Elsevier Inc. All rights reserved.

hemonc.theclinics.com

context of three patients with thrombocytopenia and the correction of the bleeding time by transfusion of whole blood. This test was normal in hemophilia. In 1918, Glanzmann[7] described a bleeding disorder characterized by a prolonged ear lobe bleeding time and normal whole blood clotting time but abnormal clot retraction.[7] In the same year, it was observed that plasma collected in oxalate would clot with the subsequent addition of calcium and the recalcification time of plasma became a common clotting test and was found to be prolonged in hemophilia. Methods were developed to measure platelets in anticoagulated whole blood using hemocytometers with large dilutions of whole blood. In 1926, von Willebrand[8] described a bleeding disorder in a family of Swedish origin in the Aland Islands, an archipelago of islands between Sweden and Finland. This disorder occurred in males and females and was characterized by easy bruising, epistaxis, menorrhagia in females, and prolonged bleeding after dental extraction. The platelet count was normal. He knew this disorder was different from hemophilia and the disorder described by Glanzmann because of the mode of inheritance (autosomal), the abnormal Duke bleeding time and the normal clot retraction. He called it pseudohemophilia.

Ten years later in New York, Quick and coworkers[9] described a test called the prothrombin time (PT). He added extract of rabbit brain to plasma, recalcified, and measured the clotting time. He considered the test an assay for prothrombin, hence the name. He found this test to be normal in hemophilia but abnormal in patients with biliary tract obstruction and concluded that prothrombin was normal in hemophilia. In 1937, it was noted that the recalcification time of hemophilic plasma was corrected by a globulin fraction and the missing clotting factor was called antihemophilic globulin.[10] Later Ivy and coworkers[11] described a variation of the ear lobe bleeding time using the volar surface of the forearm. In 1947, Pavlovsky,[12] in Buenos Aires, observed that mixing blood from two patients with hemophilia corrected the clotting time of each, thus separating two forms of hemophilia. Around the same time, Owren[13] in Norway described a female with lifelong bleeding who had a prolonged Quick PT, which was corrected with adsorbed plasma, showing that it was not a deficiency of prothrombin. This factor decayed at room temperature and was called labile factor and given the Roman numeral V, calling the disorder parahemophilia. Further mixing studies evolved with the development of the thromboplastin generation tests in 1953 by Biggs and coworkers[14,15] using adsorbed plasma and serum allowing the clear separation of hemophilia A from hemophilia B. Mixing studies subsequently identified FVII[16] (1951) and the separation of FX from FVII[17] (1956); FXI[18] (1953), FXII[19] (1953), and later other proteins of the contact phase. By 1953 an advance on the recalcification time was made by Langdell and coworkers[20] with the addition of cephalin, which became known as a "partial thromboplastin." This "partial thromboplastin" did not normalize the clotting time in hemophilia, unlike the "complete thromboplastin" used by Quick in 1935. This produced a clotting time in normal subjects of about 80 seconds. Further work by Proctor and Rapaport[21] resulted in the addition of kaolin (activator) in addition to cephalin (partial thromboplastin) resulting in the activated partial thromboplastin time (aPTT) and decreasing the clotting time to about 40 seconds. About the same time, in 1959 Hellem[22] described the property of platelet adhesion to glass beads and in 1962 Born,[23] using a modified spectrophotometer, described an optical method to assess platelet cohesion (aggregation). By 1965, coagulation laboratories had a variety of tests available to investigate bleeding disorders: the Duke or Ivy bleeding time, platelet count and morphology, tests of platelet adhesion and aggregation, the Quick PT and the aPTT, FXIII testing,[24] and mixing studies using the PT and aPTT interpretation of which is shown in **Table 1**. Even today, these tests remain the initial basis for

Table 1
Relationship between various patterns of mixing study correction and deficiency of clotting factors

	Deficient Clotting Factors	Effect of Mixing with Plasma	Mix with Adsorbed Plasma	Mix with Serum
Prolonged aPTT	FVIII; FIX FXII and other contact phase factors	Correction of clotting time	Corrected if FVIII or FXI deficiency	Corrected if FIX or FXI (or FXII) deficiency
Prolonged PT	FVII; FV FX; FII fibrinogen	Correction of clotting time	Corrected if FV (fresh plasma) or fibrinogen deficiency	Corrected if FVII or FX deficiency

testing for hereditary disorders of hemostasis. This chronologic order of events is shown in **Table 2**.

EVALUATION OF A SUSPECT INHERITED BLEEDING DISORDER

The evaluation of a patient with a suspect inherited bleeding disorder begins with a detailed personal and family bleeding history. The history should distinguish spontaneous from provoked bleeding; age of onset of bleeding; the timing of onset of bleeding if after a provocative event, such as surgery; the sites and type of bleeding (slow oozing, profuse); the duration of bleeding; concurrent medication (including

Table 2
Important chronologic events in the discovery of the clotting factors

Factor	Name	Year[a]	Reference
Factor I	Fibrinogen	1879	Hammarstem,[1] 1879
Factor II	Prothrombin	1891	Pekelharing,[2] 1891
Factor III	Tissue factor thrombokinase thromboplastin	1905	Arthus,[3] 1893
Factor IV	Calcium	1883	Owren,[13] 1947
Factor V	Labile factor		
Factor VI	Proaccelerin (FVa)		
Factor VII	Proconvertin	1951	Alexander et al,[16] 1951
Factor VIII	Antihemophilic globulin	1937	Patek & Taylor,[10] 1937
Factor IX	Christmas factor	15	
FX	Stuart-Prower factor	1956	Hougie et al,[17] 1957
FXI	Plasma antecedent factor	1953	Rosenthal et al,[18] 1953
FXII	Hageman factor	1955	Ratnoff & Colopy,[19] 1955
FXIII	Fibrin stability factor	1960	Duckert et al,[24] 1960
von Willebrand factor	FVIII:C related antigen	1971	Zimmerman et al,[28] 1971
von Willebrand factor activity	Ristocetin cofactor	1973	Weiss et al,[29] 1973

[a] Year corresponds to the description of the first patients with the disease or the factor itself.

over-the-counter drugs or herbal supplements); and the extent of bleeding (eg, whether transfusion was required as a result). Specific questioning should be made regarding easy bruising (location, frequency, size, and whether there is any known antecedent trauma), recurrent epistaxes (frequency, from one or both nostrils, duration, whether cauterization or blood transfusion was required), and excessive bleeding in association with minor trauma or surgical procedures. In the past dental extraction and tonsillectomy were more common (nowadays, wisdom teeth extraction). In females a menstrual history is required and accepting the patient's comment that her periods are "light," "moderate," or "heavy" is inadequate. The age of the menarche should be recorded and whether there was excessive bleeding at menarche and the duration of the menses. Normal menses lasts 4 to 7 days, lose on average 30 mL of blood, and the cycle length is 21 to 35 days. Specific enquiry should be made regarding the number of pads or tampons used on the heaviest days of flow, frequency of change, and the use of double protection (tampons and pads). A history of soaking a pad or tampon more frequently than once every 3 hours or soaking more than three to five pads per day for more than 1 day suggests a possible systemic bleeding disorder. The family history should make note of any known bleeding disorders with the specifics, as previously mentioned, but physicians should be wary of accepting stated diagnoses (eg, von Willebrand disease [VWD]/hemophilia) from family members because these may subsequently turn out to be misleading or erroneous. Physical examination is sometimes, but not always, helpful in clinical assessment. There are various bleeding assessment tools that consist of specific questions as previously mentioned, allowing the calculation of a score that can assist in determining the possibility of an inherited bleeding disorder.[25]

TESTS OF PRIMARY HEMOSTASIS

Patients with a defect of primary hemostasis typically give a history of mucocutaneous bleeding, easy bruising, recurrent epistaxes, menorrhagia, or bleeding after minor trauma (**Tables 3** and **4**). The initial test of primary hemostasis is a blood count to assess the cellular elements in blood, namely the white cell count, hemoglobin, and the platelet count using an automated analyzer. The mean platelet volume should be noted and the platelet histogram inspected. A Romanowsky-stained blood smear should be carefully examined to assess platelet numbers, platelet size, platelet granularity, red cells for microcytosis, and white cells for inclusions. Examples of normal platelet morphology and histogram together with a patient with a hereditary platelet disorder for comparison are shown in **Fig. 1**. Historically, the next step was to perform a skin bleeding time, but this has declined over the past 30 years. The bleeding time is performed using either lancets or a spring-loaded platform, a sphygmomanometer applied above the elbow with the pressure adjusted to 40 mm Hg. The cuts are made and the exuding blood is carefully removed by applying either gauze or filter paper to the edge of the wound, being careful not to touch the actual puncture site. Using a stopwatch, blotting occurs at 10- to 15-second intervals and the time taken for all oozing to cease is the bleeding time. The Ivy procedure is shown in **Fig. 2**. Normal bleeding time with this method is less than 9 minutes, but this is influenced by hematocrit and age. In general, bleeding times of 9 to 15 minutes are of questionable significance and greater than 20 minutes are indicative of a quantitative or qualitative platelet disorder. The problem of maintaining operator proficiency, reproducibility, and skin scarring has resulted in the abandonment of the bleeding time[26] and it has largely been replaced by an in vitro test, the Platelet Function Analyzer-100 (PFA-100, Siemens Medical Solutions USA, Malvern, PA).[27]

Table 3
Suggested sequence of testing for suspected hereditary disorders of hemostasis

	Primary Hemostasis	Secondary Hemostasis	Fibrinolysis
History	Spontaneous or provoked bleeding. Easy bruising, epistaxes, menorrhagia; prolonged bleeding, after minor injury or surgery.	Spontaneous or provoked bleeding. Bleeding into muscles or joints. Prolonged bleeding after minor injury or surgery; hematuria.	Provoked bleeding characteristic; bleeding is delayed after provocation (6–24 h). Menorrhagia. Bleeding from specific sites; gastrointestinal or genitourinary tract; oral cavity.
Primary screening tests	Platelet count and morphology. PFA-100.	aPTT. PT is less useful, but should be performed.	aPTT (for FXI deficiency). Assay of fibrinogen.
Secondary tests	Assays for von Willebrand disease and platelet function testing.	Prolonged aPTT: assays of FVIII, FIX (males); assays of FXI, FXII. Prolonged PT: assays of VII, FV, fibrinogen; assays of FX, FII.	Assay of FXI; assays of α_2-antiplasmin; assay of plasminogen.
Tertiary tests	Detailed analysis of von Willebrand factor: • Multimeric analysis • Hyporesponsiveness to low-dose ristocetin • Binding studies of FVIII:C to von Willebrand factor. • Genomic analysis of vWF gene Platelet defects: • Platelet election microscopy • Genomic analysis for platelet genes and transcription factor • Flow cytometry	Genomic analysis of FVIII and FIX genes.	Assay of thrombin activated fibrinolytic inhibitor. Assay of tissue plasminogen activator and PAI-1.

The PFA-100 measures the ability of citrated whole blood to occlude two capillary tubes lined with collagen and either ADP or epinephrine. The benchtop device is shown in **Fig. 3**. The sample is aspirated into the two separate capillary tubes and the platelets adhere to the surface, then aggregate, ultimately stopping the flow of blood. The time required (in seconds) for this to occur is called the closure time and abbreviated as collagen/ADP or collagen/epinephrine, as appropriate. Typical reference intervals are 70 to 120 seconds for collagen/ADP and 90 to 195 seconds for collagen/epinephrine. This test is frequently abnormal in VWD and hereditary functional platelet defects; however, normal closure times do not exclude these disorders, such as the milder forms of VWD and storage pool disease.[27]

The next steps in the assessment of defects in primary hemostasis are measurements of von Willebrand factor (vWF) in plasma and the performance of in vitro platelet function testing, either together or in that order. With regard to the former, the minimum testing is an immunochemical measurement of vWF antigen,[28] a functional

Table 4
Interpretation of platelet agonist using the common chemical agonists

Agonist	Response	Interpretation
ADP	Decreased or absent	Hereditary deficiency of ADP P2Y12 receptor. Glanzmann disease; such drugs as P_2Y_{12} inhibitors.
Collagen	Decreased or absent	Hereditary thrombocytopathies, such as gray platelet syndrome or Glanzmann disease.
Arachidonic	Decreased or absent	Cyclooxygenase-1 deficiency; thromboxane A_2 receptor defect.
Ristocetin	Decreased or absent	Von Willebrand disease. Bernard-Soulier syndrome.
Epinephrine	Decreased or absent	Disorder of platelet α_2-receptor; highly variable in normal patients.
Thrombin-induced dense body release	Decreased or absent	δ-Storage pool disease; release defects.

measurement of the platelet aggregating activity of vWF using ristocetin[29] (ristocetin cofactor) and the measurement of FVIII clotting activity (FVIII:C). Determination of the ABO group by reverse typing helps in interpreting these results, because levels of vWF are lower in group O patients than non-O patients. Normal levels of these analytes are typically 60% to 180%, expressed as a percentage of a normal plasma pool. A vWF antigen level of less than 30% or levels between 30% and 50% in the setting of a bleeding phenotype is diagnostic for VWD. Levels between 30% and 50% were previously classified as "low vWF": these patients may exhibit clinical bleeding, are disproportionality group O, and may benefit from treatment with desmopressin.[30] If the vWF level is less than 50%, further testing may be appropriate to determine the subtype of VWD. These tests include: vWF collagen binding activity, low levels of which suggest a lack of high-molecular-weight multimers indicating a possible type 2 VWD; multimeric analysis of plasma vWF to separate type 2A, type 2B, and type 2M; aggregometry to assess the response to ristocetin (discussed later); measurement of the binding of FVIII to vWF for type 2N; measurement of the vWF propeptide to distinguish synthetic versus clearance defects; and analysis of the vWF gene particularly with respect to Exon 28 for specific mutations. More details of these tests are beyond the scope of this article and are discussed in more detail Angela C. Weyand and Veronica H. Flood' article, "Von Willebrand Disease: Current Status of Diagnosis and Management," in this issue.

Platelet function testing is performed using whole blood collected into trisodium citrate in the standard ratio of 1:9 and is essentially an evaluation of different aspects of platelet physiology using either platelet-rich plasma (PRP) or whole blood. PRP is obtained by slow centrifugation ($270\ g \times 10$ minutes) and platelet poor plasma by hard centrifugation ($4160\ g \times 5$ minutes), some laboratories using double centrifugation to produce a "platelet-free plasma." Platelets can also be studied in whole blood, in which case the centrifugation steps are bypassed. The gold standard for assessing platelet function has been light transmission aggregometry (LTA) but this method is cumbersome to perform and is not well standardized.[31] LTA requires the collection of a large blood sample to obtain an adequate volume of PRP. Platelet aggregates are detected by a change in optical density and quantitated as the increase in light transmission, expressed as a percentage of the difference in optical density between PRP and platelet poor (autologous plasma) autologous plasma. Whole blood

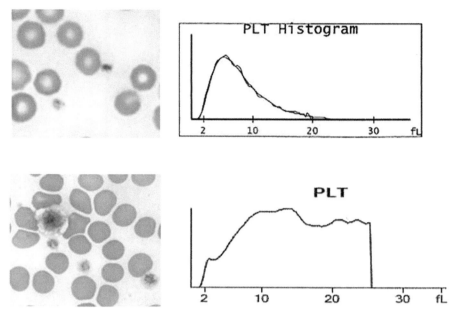

Fig. 1. Romanowsky-stained blood smear showing platelets and typical platelet histogram from a hematology analyzer. Platelets appear as small cells with internal granules, approximately one-sixth to one-third the size of red cells. The histogram shows the distribution of sizes from 2 to 28 μm. A patient with a hereditary large platelet disorder (May-Hegglin anomaly) is shown for comparison. The platelets approach the size of a red cell and the histogram is distorted and shows a right skew.

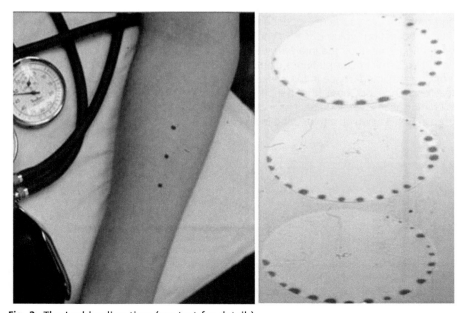

Fig. 2. The Ivy bleeding time (see text for details).

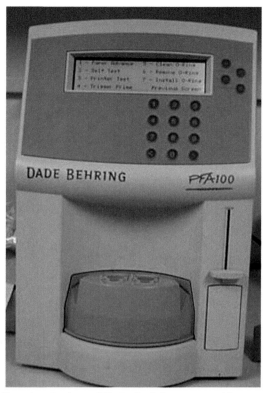

Fig. 3. The Platelet Function Analyzer-100. Each of the two cartridges uses 800 μL of citrated whole blood.

aggregometry allows the use of uncentrifuged whole blood and is performed using a smaller collection volume.[32–34] Whole blood impedance aggregometry detects platelet aggregates by the interference in the passage of a small electric current between two semicircular platinum electrodes. Platelets attach to the surface of each electrode and interference in the passage of the current is quantitated in units of electrical resistance, or Ohms. Impedance aggregometry requires adherence to a surface, which may assess an additional aspect of platelet function.[35] These changes are illustrated in **Fig. 4** in which a tube containing PRP is seen as a turbid solution, translucent

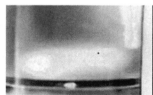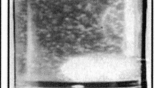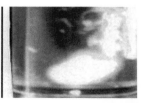

Fig. 4. Platelet aggregation. A suspension of platelet-rich plasma is seen, which appears turbid. After addition of collagen, the platelets commence to aggregate and after 2 to 3 minutes are seen as small white particulate matter. There is less turbidity, and the semicircular electrodes are clearly visible. After an additional 2 to 3 minutes, the small white particles coalesce into a larger mass and are seen attaching to the electrodes.

but not transparent. After addition of collagen, the platelets begin to aggregate and are seen as white particulate matter ("snowflakes"). The light transmission is clearly increased because it is possible to see through the suspended aggregates. As aggregation proceeds, the white particulate matter coalesces, forming a white mass ("snowball"). The white object seen at the bottom is the rotating stir bar, because platelets do not aggregate unless stirred. The whole process takes about 5 to 6 minutes for each agonist and is conducted at 37°C. The semicircular electrodes can also be visualized and the attachment of the platelet mass to the electrodes. Both LTA and whole blood impedance aggregometry require specially designed devices, a modified spectrophotometer to detect changes in turbidity and a device to measure changes in electrical resistance, respectively. Both methods produce kinetic tracings and, hence, the lag time or rate of aggregate formation as measured by the slope of the tracings is recorded. Typically, the maximum aggregation is measured (peak aggregation) but the lag time may provide useful information.[36] The slope tends to correlate with the maximum aggregation.

Platelet aggregometry is most commonly performed using a known platelet agonist, which binds to a surface receptor and causes signal response transduction using secondary messengers, which results in shape change (extrusion of cell membrane), exocytosis of dense and α-granules (secretion), surface expression of P-selectin and phosphatidylserine (activation), and exposure of a fibrinogen binding site on the glycoprotein IIB/IIIA heterodimer (facilitating aggregation). More details of the biochemistry underlying these changes are available elsewhere.[37] The agonists that are commonly used are ADP (1–10 μM), collagen (1–5 μg/mL), arachidonic acid (0.5–1 mM), thrombin (1 NIH U/mL) or TRAP (10 μM), epinephrine (10–50 μM), and ristocetin (0.1–5 mg/mL).[32–34,38,39] ADP binds to two receptors: P2Y1, which causes

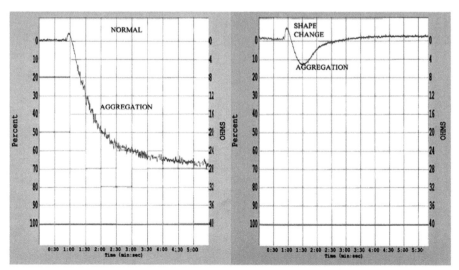

Fig. 5. Light transmission with ADP as agonist. (*Left*) Normal response: note the shape change followed by the aggregation as light transmission increases (see **Fig. 4**). (*Right*) A typical tracing as seen in the absence of the P2Y12 ADP receptor or patients on a thienopyridine. Note the preservation of the shape change and early aggregation promoted by the P2Y1 receptor but the final disaggregation as the aggregates destabilize.

shape change, some secretion, and initiates aggregation; and the P2Y12 receptor, which promotes and stabilizes the aggregates (**Fig. 5**). Collagen binds to glycoprotein VI and to a lesser extent glycoprotein Ia and is a potent aggregating and secreting agonist (**Fig. 6**). Arachidonic requires transmembrane passage where it acts as a substrate for cyclooxygenase-1, ultimately forming thromboxane A_2, which binds to thromboxane receptors and amplifies secretion and aggregation (**Fig. 7**). Epinephrine binds to α_2-receptors mediating secretion and aggregation (**Fig. 8**). Ristocetin is a positively charged chemical, which neutralizes the electrostatic repulsion between VWF and glycoprotein IB-V-IX complex, causing platelets to clump, more correctly termed agglutination (**Fig. 9**). Thrombin (or TRAP) is a potent physiologic platelet agonist, which binds to platelet PAR-2 receptors. In the illustration, only secretion is assessed (**Fig. 10**). Interpretation of abnormal responses is shown in **Table 2**. More detailed studies are beyond the scope of this article (see Frederick D. Tsai and Elisabeth M. Battinelli' article,"Inherited Platelet Disorders," in this issue. The overall approach to the investigation of defects of primary hemostasis is shown in **Table 3**.

TESTS OF SECONDARY HEMOSTASIS: IN VITRO GENERATION OF THROMBIN

Patients with a defect of secondary hemostasis give a history of bleeding into muscles or joints, and excessive bleeding with minor trauma or surgery or menorrhagia. The conventional tests used are the aPTT and the PT, respectively. These assess the so-called intrinsic and extrinsic clotting pathways, respectively. These tests are performed using citrated platelet-free plasma in automated analyzers. In the case of hereditary disorders, the aPTT is the more useful test because approximately 98% of hereditary disorders of secondary hemostasis have a clotting factor sensitive to the aPTT.

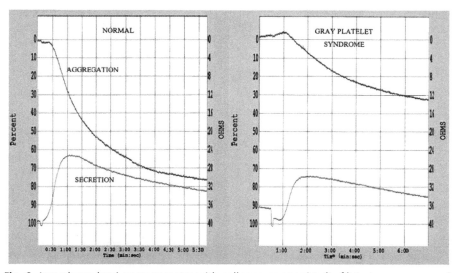

Fig. 6. Impedance lumi-aggregometry with collagen as agonist. (*Left*) A strong response is seen coupled with early secretion from the dense bodies, which precedes the detection of aggregates. (*Right*) Decreased aggregation as seen in a patient with gray platelet syndrome (α-granule deficiency) but secretion from the dense bodies is normal.

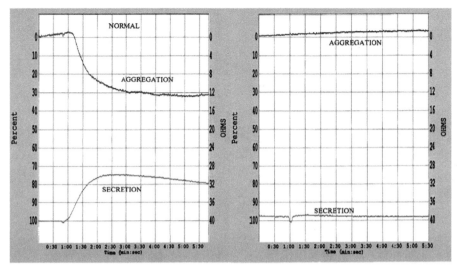

Fig. 7. Impedance lumi-aggregometry with arachidonic acid as agonist. (*Left*) A strong aggregation effect is evident, which is coincidental with dense body release. (*Right*) Typical tracing for cyclooxygenase-1 inhibition (eg, aspirin) or thromboxane A_2 receptor deficiency.

The aPTT is the current successor of the Lee-White clotting time. The difference is that it is performed in plasma; uses more defined reagents as the "partial thromboplastin," such as soybean phospholipid; and standardizes the "activator" (see history section). There are different choices of activator, largely divided into solid or "soluble" reagents. Among the solid reagents are Kaolin and micronized silica, and among the

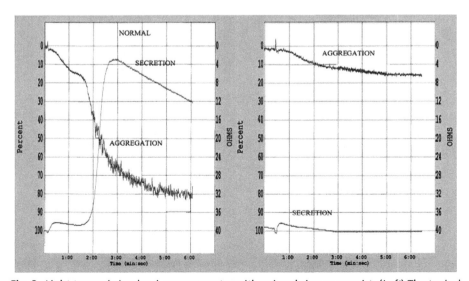

Fig. 8. Light transmission lumi-aggregometry with epinephrine as agonist. (*Left*) The typical biphasic response is evident. The secretion of dense bodies approximately coincides with the secondary wave of aggregation consistent with the released ADP facilitating larger aggregate formation. (*Right*) A diminished aggregation and secretion response to epinephrine.

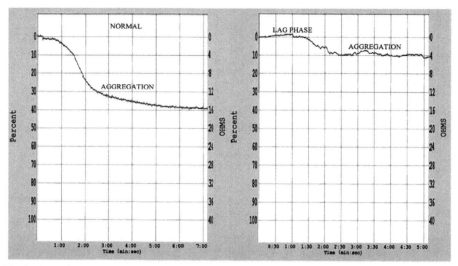

Fig. 9. Impedance aggregation to ristocetin. (*Left*) Normal. (*Right*) A patient with type 1 von Willebrand disease. Note the prolonged lag phase and decreased impedance response.

soluble reagents ellagic acid. All of these reagents share in common a negatively charged surface, which allows for the attachment of positively charged contact phase proteins, FXII, and high-molecular-weight kininogen. Because prekallikrein and FXI are carried by HMWKG, this allows close contiguity between these factors. The contact phase does not require calcium and is completed when FXI is activated to the active form (FXIa). The subsequent reaction involves the vitamin K proteins attaching to a

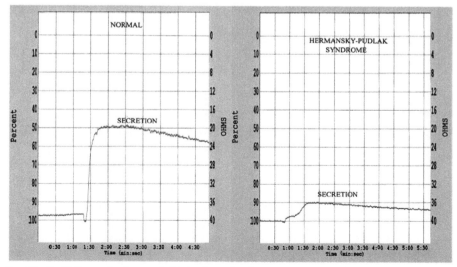

Fig. 10. (*Left*) Normal release of ATP in dense bodies in response to thrombin. (*Right*) A patient with Hermansky-Pudlak syndrome (δ-storage pool disease). ATP release is greatly diminished.

different surface (the partial thromboplastin), composed essentially of phospholipid micelles. These reagents are a mixture of negatively charged phospholipids in solution. Using calcium as a bridge, the vitamin K proteins use their negatively charged N-terminal ends to attach to the negatively charged phospholipids. FVIII and FV facilitate the generation of FXa by FIXa, and the generation of thrombin by FXa, respectively. Thus, the aPTT assesses the contact phase proteins (FXII, prekallikrein, HMWKG, and FXI), the zymogen FIX, and the regulatory proteins FV and FVIII. In general, it is much less sensitive to clotting factors lower in the cascade, such as FX, FV, FII, and fibrinogen, but hereditary deficiencies of these clotting factors are less common (FV, fibrinogen) or rare (FX,FII). aPTT reagents should have the capability to detect a reduction in FVIII only 30% or less,[40] so it is important to appreciate that an aPTT within the reference interval (normal range) does not exclude a mild contact phase deficiency or low level of FVIII or FIX.

The PT in current use is similar to the original test described by Quick (see history section) except that most clinical laboratories use recombinant tissue factor as the initiating reagent in addition to calcium. The historic reagent was called thrombokinase, then thromboplastin, which is a lipid mixture derived from mammalian lung, brain, or placenta. Recombinant human tissue factor binds to FVII, facilitating the formation of FVIIa, overcoming the inhibition by the inhibitor tissue pathway factor inhibitor, activating FX to FXa directly and subsequently the formation of thrombin. Thus, the PT assesses FVII, in particular, and the clotting factors of the so-called common pathway (FX, FV, FII), and fibrinogen.

In the past, a prolonged aPTT or PT was further studied using mixing studies in which patients' plasma was mixed with normal plasma, then retested to detect a decrease in the clotting time. A "correction" by normal plasma led to mixing studies using serum or plasma to assist in the identification of the defect (see **Table 1**). However, currently a prolonged aPTT is most efficiently studied by direct assays of FVIII and FXI in the case of females and, in addition, FIX in the case of males. A normal aPTT does not exclude minor deficiencies of these proteins, as indicated previously. A prolonged PT is most efficiently investigated by measurements of FVII, FV, and fibrinogen, because FX and FII deficiency (prothrombin) are rare (see **Table 3**). More details of these rare clotting factor deficiencies are available Glaivy Batsuli and Peter Kouides' article, "Rare Coagulation Factor Deficiencies (Factors VII, X, V, and II)," in this issue.

Clotting factors are measured using immunochemical assays (measurement of antigen) or functional assays (measurement of activity). These are typically expressed in units as percent normal, based on a standard composed of a pooled plasma from healthy human subjects, which is assigned a value of 100%, or as units per milliliter where 100% = 1 U/mL (100 U/dL). Functional assays are preferred and these are divided into two groups: chronometric (time based) assays, where the clotting factor is measured based on a modified clotting time assay using a mixing study with a plasma deficient in the clotting factor to be assayed; or chromogenic (color base) assays where the clotting factor is activated to the active enzyme, then mixed with a small chromogenic substrate (4,5 amino acid peptide), which, when cleaved, releases a colored compound. Illustrations of the principles of these assays are shown in **Fig. 11** and **Fig. 12**. Antigen assays are largely performed in reference laboratories because of the infrequency of the request in practice, but vWF antigen is routine in most coagulation laboratories and an antigenic FXIII assay is easily automated. Fibrinogen (factor I) was the first clotting factor to be described and is the clotting factor present in the highest concentration in plasma, approximately 150 to 400 mg/dL (1.5–2.0 g/L), equivalent to about 5 to 10 mM. The original assays were based on protein

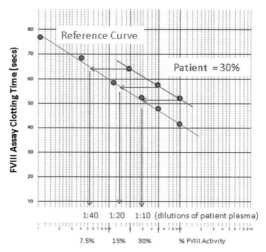

Fig. 11. Principle underlying the assays of clotting factors using the chronometric method.

chemistry and precipitation of fibrinogen by salt solutions. The most common method in widespread use worldwide is called the Clauss technique in which plasma is diluted (1:10) and then a small amount of thrombin added. The time taken for the plasma to clot is related to the fibrinogen concentration; a longer clotting time equals a lower fibrinogen concentration. This test is affected by drugs that inhibit thrombin (eg, dabigatran) but in practice the dilution effect of the plasma tends to minimize this effect. Fibrinogen is measured antigenically, commonly using an immunochemical assay, but in practice this is reserved for reference laboratories (discussed next).

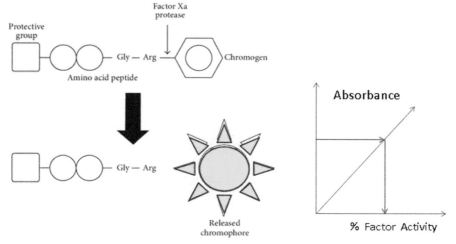

Fig. 12. Principle underlying the assay of clotting factors using the chromogenic method.

TEST OF THE FIBRINOLYTIC SYSTEM

Patients with a defect in the fibrinolytic system give a history of provoked bleeding and the typical sites are the upper aerodigestive tract or the genitourinary system. The bleeding is typically delayed, usually several hours to a day after the invasive event or provocative event. Testing for hereditary disorders of the fibrinolytic system, which cause bleeding, are frustrating and interpretation of test results challenging. The components of the fibrinolytic system are tissue plasminogen activator (or urokinase), tissue plasminogen activator inhibitor (PAI)-1 or -2, plasminogen, α_2-antiplasmin, FXI, and a carboxypeptidase U (now called thrombin activated fibrinolytic inhibitor). It is possible to measure these components in plasma but levels of tissue plasminogen activator and PAI-1 are present in low concentrations, require special collection tubes, and show diurnal variation. Assays of the other factors are technologically simpler but interpretation is difficult. In principle, low levels of α_2-antiplasmin and PAI-1 would result in unopposed fibrinolysis with bleeding. FXI is the most common of these disorders, and although commonly associated with a prolonged aPTT, should be measured directly. Bleeding caused by excessive fibrinolysis is managed by antifibrinolytics, such as tranexamic acid. More details of these disorders are available Jori E. May and colleagues' article, "Disorders of fibrinogen and fibrinolysis," in this issue.

OTHER TESTS OF HEMOSTASIS

The overall approach is shown in **Table 3**. Other less common tests performed in the hemostasis laboratory depend on the clinical history and the results of the investigations. FXIII deficiency presents as delayed bleeding or wound repair and is screened using a clot solubility test in 5M urea or 2% monochloroacetic acid or assayed immunochemically or functionally. Ari Pelcovits and colleagues' article, "Factor XIII Deficiency: A Review of Clinical Presentation and Management," in this issue. Hypofibrinogenemia, dysfibrinogenemia, and hypodysfibrinogenemia are assessed by screening tests, such as the thrombin time and the reptilase time. The thrombin time is performed by the addition of thrombin to undiluted plasma and measuring the time to clot formation. Typically, this is 18 to 24 seconds. The thrombin time is sensitive to fibrinogen concentrations but is affected by thrombin inhibitors in the plasma, such as heparins, or direct thrombin inhibitors, such as dabigatran or argatroban, or breakdown products of fibrinolysis. The reptilase time has the advantage of being insensitive to heparin. These abnormal fibrinogens are best evaluated initially by functional and antigenic measurements of fibrinogen. Typically, the antigenic level is higher than the functional level, although both are reduced. More detailed analysis requires biochemical testing or genetic testing of the various fibrinogen genes on chromosome 4 and is beyond the scope of this article (discussed in May and colleagues's article "Disorders of fibrinogen and fibrinolysis" in this issue).

CLINICS CARE POINTS

- Patients with clinical features suggestive of an hereditary disorder of hemostasis should initially have a thorough bleeding history.
- The first level of testing should be a complete blood count which includes a platelet count, mean platelet volume, blood smear examination, and performance of a PFA-100, PT, aPTT and fibrinogen level.
- If any abnormalities are found in the above screening tests, more detailed testing should be performed with clotting factor assays, assays for von Willebrand Disease and platelet function testing.

> • If no abnormalities are found, screening for FXIII deficiency or a dysfibrinogenemia should be performed.

FUNDING SOURCES

None.

ACKNOWLEDGMENTS

None.

CONFLICTS OF INTEREST

T.A. Cheves-none; J.D. Sweeney-none; S. DeMarinis -none.

REFERENCES

1. Hammarstem O. Ueber das Fibrinogen. Erster Abchnitt. Pfluegers Arch Ges Physiol 1879;19:563–622.
2. Pekelharing CA. Ueber die Bedeutung der Kalksalz fur die Gerinnung des Blutes. Int Beitr Wiss Med Virchow 1891;1:435–56.
3. Arthus M. Parallele de la coagulation du sang et de la caseification du lait. C R Soc Biol 1893;45:435–7.
4. Moraitz P. Beitrage zur Kenntnis der Blutgerinnung. Mitteilung. Deutsche Arch Klin Med 1904;79:215–33.
5. Lee RI, White PD. A clinical study of the coagulation time of blood. Am J Med Sci 1913;145:496–503.
6. Duke WW. The relation of blood platelets to hemorrhagic disease. Description of a method for determining the bleeding time and coagulation time and report of three cases of hemorrhagic disease relieved by transfusion. J Am Med Assoc 1910;55:1185–92.
7. Glanzmann E. Hereditare hamorrhogische thrombbasthenie. Ein Beitrage zur pathologie der. Blutplattchen Jahrb Kinderheilk 1918;88:1–42.
8. von Willebrand EA. Hereditär pseudohemofili. Fin Läkaresällsk Handl. 1926;68:87–112.
9. Quick AJ, Stanley-Brown M, Bancroft FW. A study of the coagulation defect in heamophilia and in jaundice. Am J Med Sci 1935;190:501–11.
10. Patek AJ, Taylor FHL. Hemophilia II. Some properties of a substance obtained from normal human plasma effective in accelerating the coagulation of hemophilic blood. J Clin Invest 1937;16:113–24.
11. Ivy AC, Nelson D, Bucher G. The standardization of certain factors in the cutaneous venostasis bleeding time technique. J Lab Clin Med 1941;26:1812–22.
12. Pavlovsky A. Contribution to the pathogenesis of hemophilia. Blood 1947;2:185–91.
13. Owren PA. Parahaemophilia: a haemorrhagic diathesis due to absence of a previously unknown clotting factor. Lancet 1947;1:446–8.
14. Biggs R, Douglas AS. The thromboplastin generation test. J Clin Pathol 1953;6:23–9.
15. Biggs R, Douglas AS, Macfarlane RG, et al. Christmas disease: a condition previously mistaken for haemophilia. Br Med J 1952;2:1378–82.

16. Alexander B, Goldstein R, Landwehr G, et al. Congenital SPCA deficiency: a hithererto unrecognized coagulation defect with hemorrhage rectified by serum and serum fractions. J Clin Invest 1951;30:596–608.
17. Hougie C, Barrow EM, Graham JB. Stuart clotting defect. I Segregation of a hereditary hemorrhagic state from the heterogenous group heretofore called "stable factor" (SPCA), proconvertin, factor VII) deficiency. J Clin Invest 1957;36:485–96.
18. Rosenthal RL, Dreskin OH, Rosenthal N. New hemophilia-like disease caused by deficiency of a third plasma thromboplastin factor. Proc Soc Exp Biol Med 1953; 1:171–4.
19. Ratnoff OD, Colopy JE. A familial hemorrhagic trait associated with a deficiency of clot-promoting fraction of plasma. J Clin Invest 1955;34:602–14.
20. Langdell RD, Wagner RH, Brinkhaus KM. Effect of antihemophilic factor on one stage clotting tests. A presumptive test for hemophilia and a simple one stage antihemophilic factor assay procedure. J Lab Clin Med 1953;41:637–47.
21. Proctor RR, Rapaport SI. The partial thromboplastin time with kaolin. A simple screening test for the first stage plasma clotting factor deficiencies. Am Clin Pathol 1961;36:12–219.
22. Hellem J. The adhesiveness of human blood platelets in vitro. Scand J Clin Lab Invest 1960;12:1–117.
23. Born GVR. Aggregation of blood platelet by adenosine diphosphate and its reversal. Nature (London) 1962;194:927–9.
24. Duckert F, Jung E, Shmerling DH. A hitherto undescribed congenital haemorrhagic diathesis probably due to fibrin stabilizing factor deficiency. Thromb Diath Haemorrh 1960;5:179–86.
25. Rydz N, James PD. The evolution and value of bleeding assessment tools. J Thromb Haemost 2012;10:2223–9.
26. Rodgers RP, Levin J. A critical reappraisal of the bleeding time. Semin Thromb Haemost 1990;16:1–20.
27. Harrison P, Robinson M, Liesher R, et al. The PFA-100: a potential screening tool for the assessment of platelet dysfunction. Clin Lab Haematol 2002;24:225–32.
28. Zimmerman TS, Ratnoff OD, Powell AE. Immunologic differentiation of classic hemophilia (factor VIII deficiency) and von Willebrand's disease. J Clin Invest 1971; 50:244–54.
29. Weiss HJ, Hager LW, Rickles FR, et al. Quantitative assay of a plasma factor deficient in von Willebrand's disease that is necessary for platelet aggregation. Relationship to factor VIII procoagulant activity and antigen content. J Clin Invest 1973;52:2708–16.
30. Lavin M, O'Donnell JS. How I treat low von Willebrand factor levels. Blood 2019; 133:795–804.
31. Cattaneo M, Hayward CP, Moffat KA, et al. Results of a worldwide survey on the assessment of platelet function by light transmission aggregometry: a report from the platelet physiology subcommittee of the SSC of the ISTH. J Thromb Haemost 2009;7:1029.
32. Sweeney JD, Labuzetta JW, Fitzpatrick JE. The effect of the platelet count on the aggregation response and adenosine triphosphate release in an impedance lumi-aggregometer. Am J Clin Pathol 1988;89:655–9.
33. Sweeney JD, Hoernig LA, Michnik A, et al. Whole blood aggregometry. Influence of sample collection and delay in study performance on test results. Am J Clin Pathol 1989;92:676–9.
34. Sweeney JD, Labuzetta JW, Michielson CE, et al. Whole blood aggregation using impedance and particle counter methods. Am J Clin Pathol 1989;92:794–7.

35. Sweeney JD, Labuzetta JW, Bernstein ZP, et al. Ristocetin induced platelet aggregate formation and adherence to the probe of an impedance aggregometer. Am J Clin Pathol 1990;93:548–51.

36. Sweeney JD, Hoernig LA, Fitzpatrick JE. Whole blood aggregation in von Willebrand disease. Am J Hematol 1989;32:190–3.

37. Rao AK, Gabbeta J. Congenital disorders of platelet signal transduction. Arterioscler Thromb Vasc Biol 2000;20:285–9.

38. Hayward CPM, Pai M, Liu Y, et al. Diagnostic utility of light transmission platelet aggregometry: results from a prospective study of individuals referred for bleeding disorder assessments. J Thromb Haemost 2009;7:676–84.

39. Philipp CS, Dilley A, Miller CH, et al. Platelet functional defects in women with unexplained menorrhagia. J Thromb Haemost 2003;1:477–84.

40. Bowyer A, Kitchen S, Makris M. The responsiveness of different APTT reagents to mild factor VIII, IX and XI deficiencies. Int J Lab Hematol 2011;33:154–8.

Primary Hemostasis/Platelet Disorders

Inherited Platelet Disorders

Frederick D. Tsai, MD, PhD[a,b,c], Elisabeth M. Battinelli, MD, PhD[a,c],*

KEYWORDS

- Platelets • Bleeding • Inherited platelet disorders

KEY POINTS

- An inherited platelet disorder should be suspected in patients with mucocutaneous bleeding or periprocedural hemorrhage in the absence of secondary causes and a suggestive family history.
- Defects in platelet aggregation and activation can occur at the level of platelet receptors, platelet signaling, platelet granule release, platelet cytoskeletal remodeling, and platelet hematopoiesis.
- Clinical history and laboratory analysis of platelet morphology and aggregation in response to specific agonists can be used to narrow the differential diagnosis when an inherited platelet disorder is suspected.
- Management of inherited platelet disorders is primarily supportive, with platelet transfusions and antifibrinolytic therapy.
- Awareness and education in patients with an inherited platelet disorder is critical to prevent future occurrences of bleeding.

CASE VIGNETTE

A 23-year-old woman with a history of epistaxis and gingival bleeding as a child and heavy menses presents with abnormal uterine bleeding after stopping her oral contraceptive. She is on no other medications. She has a normal platelet count, prothrombin time, activated partial thromboplastin time, and fibrinogen. Thrombin time is normal, and a von Willebrand panel is sent and is also normal. Platelet aggregation studies are performed and are abnormal, raising concern for a congenital platelet disorder.

[a] Division of Hematology, Department of Medicine, Brigham and Women's Hospital, 75 Francis St, Boston, MA 02115, USA; [b] Division of Hematologic Neoplasia, Department of Medical Oncology, Dana-Farber Cancer Institute, 450 Brookline Avenue, Boston, MA 02215, USA; [c] Harvard Medical School, 25 Shattuck St, Boston, MA 02115, USA
* Corresponding author. Division of Hematology, Brigham and Women's Hospital, 4 Blackfan Circle, 7th floor, Boston, MA 02115, USA
E-mail address: embattinelli@bwh.harvard.edu

Hematol Oncol Clin N Am 35 (2021) 1069–1084
https://doi.org/10.1016/j.hoc.2021.07.003
0889-8588/21/© 2021 Elsevier Inc. All rights reserved.

hemonc.theclinics.com

INTRODUCTION

Bleeding disorders are a common hematologic complication affecting patients. Impairments in either of the 2 necessary components for clot formation, platelets, and coagulation factors can lead to ineffective hemostasis. Abnormal bleeding due to platelet dysfunction typically presents with mucocutaneous bleeding and delayed hemostasis or hemorrhage following surgical procedures or trauma. Although acquired causes of platelet dysfunction are more common, an inherited platelet disorder should be suspected in patients with a presentation or bleeding history consistent with abnormal platelet function, lack of secondary causes, such as medication effect or a systemic process, and a familial history of similar bleeding suggestive of a congenital disorder. This review outlines the inherited disorders of platelet function and the biological basis for their pathophysiology.

PLATELET ACTIVATION

The interaction of platelets with the coagulation cascade to initiate hemostasis is a multistep, coordinated process involving receptor activation, intracellular signaling and cytoskeletal remodeling, and granule release.[1]

On injury to blood vessels, endothelial damage exposes collagen fibrils from the subendothelial space, which binds to circulating von Willebrand factor (VWF). Interaction of VWF with the glycoprotein Ib-IX-V complex (GPIb/IX) leads to initial platelet adhesion at these sites of injury. Subsequent interaction of platelet receptors with other exposed proteins in the subendothelial matrix triggers the activation of multiple signaling cascades, which results in release of platelet granules. The cargo proteins stored within each granule type (ADP and serotonin from dense granules, and fibrinogen, VWF, and coagulation factors from alpha granules) further promote platelet activation and coagulation in a positive feedback mechanism. Granule secretion and fusion with the platelet plasma membrane also serves to increase platelet surface area and uncover additional surface receptors involved in aggregation. These processes accelerate the local recruitment of other platelets, which bind to each other through the interaction of fibrinogen with the glycoprotein IIb-IIIa complex (GPIIb/IIIa). Activated platelets also undergo cytoskeletal remodeling with rapid polymerization of cytoplasmic actin, increasing structural cohesion of the newly formed platelet plug. The platelet plug serves as a platform for thrombin activation through the coagulation cascade, allowing for fibrin crosslinking and stabilization of the incipient clot.

Defects at each step of platelet aggregation and activation have been described both genetically and phenotypically, allowing for elucidation of specific aspects of platelet biology and accounting for the bleeding presentations in affected patents.[2] As such, the inherited platelet disorders can be broadly classified as affecting platelet receptors, platelet signaling, platelet granule release, platelet cytoskeletal structure, and platelet hematopoiesis and maturation (**Fig. 1**). These are reviewed as follows.

PLATELET RECEPTOR DEFECTS

The cell surface of platelets contains integrins, transmembrane glycoprotein complexes that mediate adhesion and aggregation to VWF, collagen, and other platelets, and G protein-coupled receptors that respond to extracellular agonists, including epinephrine, ADP, thromboxane, and thrombin, and activate signal transduction pathways. Decreased expression or impaired function of these receptors from congenital mutations can result in defective platelet binding or activation, preventing initiation of hemostasis.

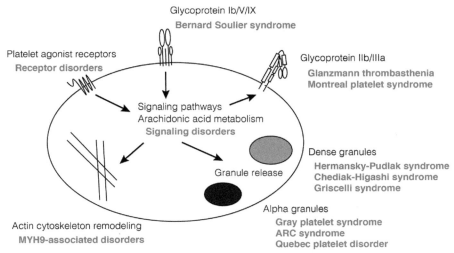

Fig. 1. Components of platelet activation and associated disorders. Platelet activation begins with glycoprotein Ib/V/IX complex binding to injured epithelium via interaction with VWF. Platelet adhesion and agonist signaling through G protein-coupled receptors induce signaling pathways and arachidonic acid metabolism, resulting in unfolding of glycoprotein IIb/IIIa and fibrinogen binding, actin cytoskeleton remodeling and platelet shape change, and secretion of dense and alpha granules. Representative disorders of each of these steps are indicated in bold.

Bernard-Soulier Syndrome

First described in 1948, the Bernard-Soulier syndrome (BSS) describes deficiency in the GPIb/IX complex on platelets leading to thrombocytopenia and bleeding diathesis. Classic BSS is an autosomal recessive disorder characterized by mutations in any of the 3 genes, GP1A, GP1B, and GP9, that encode for the components of the GPIb/IX complex.[3] Loss of platelet GPIb/IX complex formation results in compromised binding of platelets to VWF and lack of platelet adhesion. Clinically, patients present with a moderately decreased platelet count and large platelet size on peripheral smear. Clinical bleeding is often disproportionate to the degree of thrombocytopenia. Mechanistically, BSS resembles von Willebrand disease, with platelet aggregation studies demonstrating decreased response and lack of platelet agglutination to ristocetin, but otherwise preserved response to ADP, epinephrine, thrombin, and collagen. BSS can be distinguished from von Willebrand disease by the presence of normal VWF and factor VIII levels, and an inability of exogenous VWF to overcome patient bleeding. Flow cytometry of platelets shows decreased platelet surface GPIb receptors.

Monoallelic forms of BSS have been described as a frequent cause of mild macrothrombocytopenia, with single allele variants in GPIBA and GPIBB identified by whole exome sequencing.[4,5] An autosomal dominant form, the Bolzano variant (p.A172V in GPIBA), has also been described and is thought to be responsible for a regional variant of BSS, Mediterranean macrothrombocytopenia.[6]

Glanzmann Thrombasthenia

Defects in the platelet integrin complex GPIIb/IIIa (also known as integrin α2b-β3) lead to the rare autosomal recessive disorder Glanzmann thrombasthenia.[7] Qualitative or quantitative defects in GPIIb/IIIa result in inability of platelets to bind to fibrinogen, which is required for platelet aggregation in response to all physiologic agonists. This presents as severe mucocutaneous bleeding due to inability to form platelet plugs. Platelet aggregation tests in these patients show marked decrease or absence of platelet aggregation in response to all platelet agonists, except for ristocetin. The shape change response of platelets is preserved, and although platelet dense granule secretion is decreased, thrombin activation induces normal granule secretion. Flow cytometry demonstrates decreased platelet surface GPIIb/IIIa. Glanzmann thrombasthenia is clinically similar to congenital afibrinogenemia, although is distinguished by preserved clotting times and normal fibrinogen levels.

Mutations in *FERMT3* and *RASGRP2* have been described in patients with similar clinical presentations and platelet impairments to Glanzmann thrombasthenia.[8] Mutations in *FERMT3* are associated with leukocyte adhesion deficiency type III, which presents clinically in infancy with abnormal wound healing, increased infection, and severe bleeding.[9,10] Similarly, mutations in *RASGRP2* present early in life and demonstrate abnormal platelet aggregation.[11–13] Both FERMT3 and RasGRP2 are cytoplasmic proteins implicated in integrin activation, and dysfunctional "inside-out" signaling is thought to account for the Glanzmann-like phenotype seen in these patients.

Montreal Platelet Syndrome

The Montreal platelet syndrome was first observed in individuals of French-Canadian descent, and phenotypically presents as an inherited macrothrombocytopenia with overlapping features of type 2B von Willebrand disease. Individuals with Montreal platelet syndrome have heterozygous VWF p.V1316M mutations, and clinically present with severe thrombocytopenia, mucocutaneous bleeding, and giant platelets.[14] Similar to that seen in other platelet receptor disorders, essential signaling requirements for GPIIb/IIIa integrin activation are lost in Montreal platelet syndrome.[15]

Signaling Receptor Defects

Various physiologic agonists interact with receptors on platelet surfaces, inducing numerous signal transduction pathways as part of platelet activation. These receptors include G protein-coupled receptors that interact with epinephrine, ADP, platelet-activating factor, thrombin, and thromboxane.[16] Glycoprotein Ia/IIa (also known as integrin α2-β1) and glycoprotein VI on platelet surfaces interact with collagen and induce both adhesion and platelet granule secretion. Deficiencies in surface receptors to ADP, collagen, epinephrine, and thromboxane A2 have been described, resulting in impaired platelet aggregation and/or secretion from their specific agonists.[17] These can be measured with platelet aggregation assays showing blunted response to exogenous agonists when performed in vitro.

PLATELET SIGNALING DEFECTS

The series of signaling cascades triggered by platelet agonist–receptor interaction leads to platelet activation and granule secretion, which in turn causes a positive feedback loop by releasing further agonists to augment hemostasis. Secreted ADP from dense granules acts on platelet surface receptors P2Y1 and P2Y12, activating adenylyl cyclase and protein kinase C effector pathways. Calcium-mediated activity of phospholipase A2 and arachidonic acid metabolism and signaling are also increased. The plasma membrane of activated platelets undergoes dynamic change, with exposure of negatively charged phospholipid surfaces on the outer leaflet creating a platform for coagulation factors to bind and associate, leading to extracellular thrombin activation through the coagulation cascade. Defects in platelet signal transduction have been described not only at the level of specific receptors but also downstream at intracellular effectors.

Cyclooxygenase Deficiency and Arachidonic Acid Metabolism

Intracellular calcium signaling activates phospholipase C and phospholipase A2, which generate arachidonic acid from phospholipids. Arachidonic acid metabolism is a central pathway in response to platelet activation and through the activity of cyclooxygenase and thromboxane synthase culminates in synthesis of thromboxane A2. Thromboxane A2 is a potent platelet agonist that plays multiple roles in hemostasis, including platelet aggregation, platelet granule secretion, and vasoconstriction. Patients with congenital deficiencies of phospholipase A2, cyclooxygenase, and thromboxane synthase have been described to have abnormal platelet aggregation and secretion, presenting with variable bleeding.[17] Platelet aggregation assays in these patients resemble those seen in secondary platelet disorders due to medication effects from aspirin, nonsteroidal anti-inflammatory agents (NSAIDs), or other drugs that inhibit cyclooxygenase. As such, patients with inherited deficiencies in these enzymes can be diagnosed only in the absence of exogenous medication use.

Scott Syndrome

Platelet activation results in active reorganization of phospholipids in the lipid membrane.[18] Under resting conditions, phospholipids are distributed and maintained asymmetrically between the inner and outer leaflets of the lipid bilayer, with the negatively charged phospholipid phosphatidylserine primarily confined to the cytoplasmic inner leaflet. On platelet activation, intracellular calcium signaling results in randomization of lipids and loss of asymmetry, with the membrane protein scramblase transporting phospholipids between the 2 lipid leaflets. Exposure of phosphatidylserine on the extracellular outer leaflet of platelet membranes creates an anionic platform on platelet surfaces that favors interaction and binding of coagulation factors with plasma calcium ions, allowing for assembly of the tenase and prothrombinase complexes. Defects in scramblase activity lead to a rare bleeding disorder named Scott syndrome,[19] in which loss of phosphatidylserine exposure on platelet surfaces results in impaired coagulation activity and moderate to severe bleeding. Patients have normal platelet structure, secretion, and aggregation, normal bleeding times, and normal coagulation factors, although Scott syndrome platelets fail to promote fibrin formation, and activation of the prothrombinase and tenase complexes are prolonged in response to Russell's viper venom.[18]

PLATELET GRANULE DISORDERS

Mature platelets contain 3 types of secretory granules: dense granules, alpha granules, and lysosomes. Defective granule formation or secretion is the hallmark of the class of platelet disorders known as storage pool disorders, which manifest as bleeding diathesis, prolonged bleeding times, and platelet functional studies showing impairment in secretion. The biogenesis and sorting of specific protein cargo to their respective granules is a tightly regulated process, and genetic disorders in these pathways can result in impaired secretion of dense granules, alpha granules, or both.

Dense Granule Storage Pool Disorders

Platelet dense granules are related to lysosomes and originate from the endosomal system.[20] They primarily contain phosphate, ADP, and serotonin, and cargo release promotes and accelerates platelet aggregation.[21] Dense granule storage pool disorders present with variable severity but typically a mild to moderate bleeding diathesis, and on platelet aggregation studies have impaired response to low-level agonists including collagen, ADP, and epinephrine, and a blunted to absent secondary aggregation curve.

The Hermansky-Pudlak syndrome (HPS) is an autosomal recessive dense granule storage pool disorder that clinically presents with bleeding, oculocutaneous albinism, congenital nystagmus, decreased visual acuity, granulomatous colitis, and pulmonary fibrosis.[22] Ten genetically distinct subtypes have been described: the 10 HPS gene products are ubiquitously expressed and are critical in trafficking to lysosome-related organelles, including platelet dense granules and melanosomes. The cellular defects in HPS cause lysosomal accumulation of ceroid lipofuscin, leading to the clinical phenotype of oculocutaneous albinism; the mechanism of pulmonary fibrosis is not clearly understood. Although described worldwide, HPS has increased prevalence in Puerto Rico due to founder mutations in *HPS1* and *HPS3*, with 1 in 21 persons as a carrier of *HPS1* and 1 in 1800 persons having HPS-1 in northwest Puerto Rico.[23]

Other genetic impairments in lysosomal trafficking result in dense granule impairment. Chediak-Higashi syndrome, caused by mutations in the *LYST* gene (lysosomal trafficking regulator), results in giant cytoplasmic inclusions in leukocytes and absent dense granules in platelets.[24,25] An autosomal recessive disorder with fewer than 500 cases worldwide, Chediak-Higashi syndrome clinically presents with mild bleeding, partial oculocutaneous albinism, and recurrent pyogenic infections due to dysfunction of cytotoxic T and NK cells.[26] Griscelli syndrome, characterized by mutations in *MYO5A* (myosin VA) and *RAB27A*, has also been described as a cause of decreased platelet dense granules in affected individuals.[27–29]

Alpha Granule Storage Pool Disorders

Alpha granules are the most abundant platelet granules and are derived from budding of small vesicles from the trans-Golgi network.[30] Their cargo consists of both membrane proteins that are exposed on platelet surfaces during platelet activation, including integrins and immunoglobulin receptors, and soluble proteins and coagulation factors, including VWF, fibrinogen, inactive precursors of thrombin and prothrombin, and high molecular weight kininogens.[31] Release of alpha granule contents during platelet activation accelerates coagulation, as well as mediating other processes, including inflammation, angiogenesis, wound healing, and host defense.

Inherited defects in alpha granule biogenesis include the gray platelet syndrome and the arthrogryposis-renal dysfunction-cholestasis (ARC) syndrome. The gray platelet syndrome is so named as phenotypically, platelets appear large and agranular on peripheral smear.[32] Patients present with mild thrombocytopenia, prolonged bleeding times, and a variable bleeding diathesis. Different genetic alterations have been described for gray platelet syndrome, and the exact mechanisms are not fully understood. Autosomal recessive forms of gray platelet syndrome occur with mutations in *NBEAL2*, a scaffolding protein found in mechanistic studies to have a critical role in development of alpha granules, as well as roles in immunity and neutrophil structure.[33,34] Autosomal dominant inheritance of gray platelet syndrome has been described in association with mutations in the transcription factor *GFI1B*, which regulates hematopoiesis and the differentiation of megakaryocytes.[35] X-linked associations of gray platelet syndrome have also been seen in patients with *GATA1* mutations, which is thought to have a downstream effect on regulation of *NBEAL2* transcription similar to the autosomal recessive form.[36]

Mutations in the *VPS33B* gene, a membrane-associated protein that regulates assembly and fusion of vesicles from the trans-Golgi network and associates with alpha granules, result in the ARC syndrome.[30] Variants in *VPS16B* have also been described. Patients with ARC have platelets with absent alpha granules, although platelet count and size are otherwise normal. Congenital limb malformations, renal tubular dysfunction and nephrogenic diabetes insipidus, and neonatal cholestasis also characterize this syndrome.

The Quebec platelet disorder is an autosomal dominant storage pool disorder characterized by abnormal proteolysis of alpha granule proteins and that presents with delayed bleeding.[37] Tandem duplication of chromosome 10 leads to duplication of the *PLAU* gene (platelet urokinase-type plasminogen activator), which becomes overexpressed in megakaryocytes and leads to premature proteolytic degradation of alpha granule proteins.[38,39] Although platelet counts are normal to reduced, platelet functional studies show impairment with a defective aggregation response to epinephrine.

PLATELET CYTOSKELETAL STRUCTURE DEFECTS

Platelet production begins in the bone marrow, where megakaryocytes differentiate and develop from hematopoietic stem and precursor cells in response to thrombopoietin (**Fig. 2**). Megakaryocytes increase in size and become polyploid as they mature, forming granules that assemble through a process involving changes to megakaryocyte cell structure and cytoplasmic organization. Dynamic remodeling of the actin cytoskeleton creates elongated branches and extrusions called proplatelets, which then fission into individual platelets with cytoskeletons composed of cytoplasmic actin filaments and membrane skeleton proteins. These cytoskeleton dynamics are dependent on myosin and β-tubulin,[40,41] and defects in both lead to

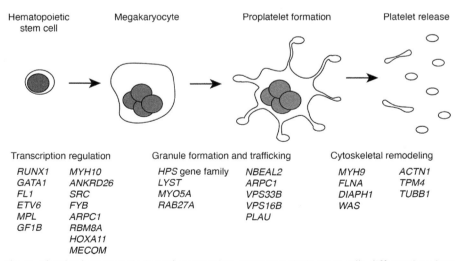

Hematopoietic stem cell		Megakaryocyte	Proplatelet formation		Platelet release	

Transcription regulation		Granule formation and trafficking		Cytoskeletal remodeling	
RUNX1	MYH10	HPS gene family	NBEAL2	MYH9	ACTN1
GATA1	ANKRD26	LYST	ARPC1	FLNA	TPM4
FL1	SRC	MYO5A	VPS33B	DIAPH1	TUBB1
ETV6	FYB	RAB27A	VPS16B	WAS	
MPL	ARPC1		PLAU		
GF1B	RBM8A				
	HOXA11				
	MECOM				

Fig. 2. Platelet hematopoiesis and maturation. Hematopoietic stem cells differentiate into megakaryocytes in response to thrombopoietin signaling and changes to epigenetic and transcriptional programming. Megakaryocytes undergo multiple nuclear divisions, form granules, and remodel their actin cytoskeleton to form elongated protrusions called proplatelets, which in turn fission into numerous platelets. Genes implicated in congenital platelet disorders involving these steps are listed.

congenital macrothrombocytopenias and bleeding disorders with impaired platelet maturation and defective clot formation and stability.

MYH9-Associated Disorders: the May-Hegglin Anomaly

The May-Hegglin anomaly is the prototype of a class of syndromes including Fechtner, Sebastian, and Epstein syndromes, all of which originate from mutations in *MYH9*.[40] *MYH9* encodes myosin heavy chain, which mediates intracellular contractile forces and actin cytoskeleton, and mutations in *MYH9* have been described throughout the gene, leading to loss of function. Affected megakaryocytes have reduced migration to the vascular sinus, altered formation of platelets, and ectopic and reduced platelet release into the marrow.[42] Clinically, this presents as large platelets with typically normal platelet function but reduced clot stability due to defects in platelet cytoskeleton dynamics. Peripheral blood smears are notable for a macrothrombocytopenia and Döhle body-like inclusions in neutrophils. Disorders in *MYH9* are associated with other syndromic manifestations including sensorineural hearing loss, early cataracts, progressive glomerulonephritis, and elevated liver enzymes.

Mutations in other genes involved in cytoskeletal maintenance have been described, all of which have autosomal dominant inheritance, syndromic phenotypes similar to that of *MYH9*-related disease, and variable degrees of thrombocytopenia and bleeding. Mutations in *FLNA*, which encodes filamin, are associated with an X-linked macrothrombocytopenia and other developmental defects, including Ehlers-Danlos syndrome.[43] Filamin is thought to play a role in GPIIb/IIIa signaling.[44] These patients have large, fragile platelets that are rapidly removed from circulation, leading to macrothrombocytopenia and severe bleeding.[45,46] Mutations in *DIAPH1*, a member of the formin family that regulates actin filament formation and microtubule assembly, similarly result in a bleeding diathesis and sensorineural hearing loss.[47] Affected megakaryocytes have reduced and premature proplatelet formation, as seen in *MYH9*-related disease. Inherited thrombocytopenias have also been described with mutations in *ACTN1* (α-actinin), *TPM4* (tropomyosin), and *TUBB1* (β-tubulin),[41,48] all of which present with moderate thrombocytopenias and variable bleeding phenotypes.[49]

DISORDERS OF PLATELET HEMATOPOIESIS AND MATURATION

The differentiation of hematopoietic stem and precursor cells into megakaryocytes occurs under careful epigenetic and transcription control.[50] Dysregulation of these transcription programs can lead to impaired platelet hematopoiesis, resulting in thrombocytopenias and bleeding diatheses, although clinical manifestations of these congenital disorders are often multisystemic and present in advance of a clinical bleeding syndrome.

Paris-Trousseau Syndrome and Associated Disorders of Megakaryopoiesis

The Paris-Trousseau/Jacobsen syndrome is an autosomal dominant macrothrombocytopenia with giant platelets containing fused alpha granules that can be readily seen on morphology. Patients have other syndromic presentations including psychomotor retardation and facial and cardiac abnormalities.[51] Affected individuals were found to have deletion of chromosome 11q23 to 24, with the causative gene identified as *FL1* (friend leukemia integration 1), an ETS transcription factor that acts as a main regulator of megakaryopoiesis and controls genes including *MPL*, *GPIBA*, and *ITGA2*.[52] Megakaryocytes demonstrate prolonged expression of the cytoskeletal protein *MYH10*, resulting in immature megakaryocytes that fail to differentiate properly.[53] Autosomal recessive variants of *FL1* result in a Paris-Trousseau platelet phenotype, without the cardiac or developmental abnormalities associated with the autosomal dominant syndrome.

Similar presentations can be seen with other inherited mutations in genes that regulate megakaryopoiesis.[50] Patients with *ETV6*-associated thrombocytopenia harbor mutations in the tumor suppressor gene *ETV6*, which functions similarly to *FL1*.[54–56] This autosomal dominant condition, which confers predisposition to acute lymphoblastic leukemia, clinically presents with moderate thrombocytopenia and defective platelet interactions with fibrinogen, but mild to no bleeding. Mutations in *SRC*,[57–59] *FYB*,[60,61] and *ARPC1*[62] have also been described, with microthrombocytopenia and variable bleeding.

Familial platelet disorder with predisposition to acute myeloid leukemia (FPD-AML) is an autosomal dominant disorder characterized by mutations in the hematopoietic master regulator *RUNX1*.[63–65] This syndrome presents with variable penetrance but is associated with defective platelet function, reduced dense granule secretion, and variable bleeding.[66] *RUNX1* regulates the synthesis of numerous platelet proteins and represses expression of *MYH10* and *ANKRD26* in immature megakaryocytes similarly to *FL1*; loss of *RUNX1* silencing of *MYH10* and *ANKRD26* thus contributes to failure of megakaryocyte differentiation. Inherited mutations in *ANKRD26* have also been described in familial thrombocytopenias. These mutations occur in the 5′ untranslated region of *ANKRD26* and prevent its downregulation by *RUNX1* and *FL1*, leading to a moderate thrombocytopenia with mild bleeding, and platelets of normal size but with decreased density of glycoprotein Ia/IIa receptors and decreased alpha granules.[67–69]

Wiskott-Aldrich syndrome (WAS), originally described as eczema-thrombocytopenia-immunodeficiency syndrome, arises from mutations in the *WAS* gene on Xp11.23, which was further characterized as a regulator of the actin cytoskeleton in hematopoietic cells. Affected individuals present with severe microthrombocytopenia, immunodeficiencies, eczema, and predisposition to autoimmune conditions and malignancy.[70] Life-threatening hemorrhage can occur as a consequence of thrombocytopenia.[71] The mechanism of platelet dysfunction is thought to be due to impaired hematopoiesis and increased peripheral autoantibody-mediated destruction, although a recent cohort study of patients with WAS demonstrated a hyperactivated platelet phenotype with derangements in platelet structure and aggregation response.[72] Beyond supportive transfusions, splenectomy and allogeneic hematopoietic stem cell transplantation are the primary modalities of treatment.

Congenital Amegakaryocytic Thrombocytopenia

Severe thrombocytopenia is seen in congenital amegakaryocytic thrombocytopenia (CAMT), a rare bone marrow failure syndrome characterized by mutations in the thrombopoietin receptor gene, *MPL*, resulting in failure of megakaryocytic differentiation.[73] Bone marrow biopsies demonstrate isolated absence of megakaryocytes and complete loss of platelet production. Allogeneic stem cell transplantation is the primary treatment modality.

Congenital Malformation Syndromes

Although they share common findings of absent megakaryopoiesis and severe thrombocytopenia, in contrast to CAMT, other skeletal and developmental abnormalities are seen in thrombocytopenia-absent radius (TAR) syndrome and radioulnar synostosis with amegakaryocytic thrombocytopenia (RUSAT). TAR syndrome is associated with bilateral radius aplasia and developmental defects, and reduced response to thrombopoietin.[74,75] Whole exome sequencing of affected patients revealed loss of heterozygosity of *RBM8A*; microdeletion of chromosome 1.21.1 containing the *RBM8A* gene was accompanied by rare single nucleotide polymorphisms on the regulatory region of *RBM8A* on the second allele, leading to loss of function of *RBM8A*.[76] The role of RBM8A and its mechanism in causing TAR syndrome remains largely unknown. In RUSAT, an autosomal dominant syndrome, heterozygous truncating mutations in *HOXA11* lead to skeletal defects and amegakaryocytosis.[77,78] An autosomal recessive variant has been described with de novo missense mutations in *MECOM*, encoding the transcription factor EVI1 that has been implicated in cell cycle and terminal differentiation of hematopoietic stem and progenitor cells.[79]

DIAGNOSIS AND MANAGEMENT

Clinical workup for a suspected inherited platelet disorder begins with the patient history. Signs and symptoms of mucocutaneous bleeding and delayed hemostasis or hemorrhage following surgical procedures or trauma suggest a platelet origin of bleeding, and family history of similar bleeding can suggest specific inheritance patterns. A careful review of medications and medical comorbidities is needed to determine whether an acquired or secondary platelet disorder could be present, with common culprits including antiplatelet agents such as aspirin or NSAIDs. Aspects of the patient history that indicate multisystem involvement or developmental features might be consistent with a specific congenital syndrome and should heighten the clinician's concern.

Laboratory workup should include a comprehensive blood count and manual review of the peripheral smear to assess platelet morphology. Notable features from the peripheral blood smear include platelet number, size, and granular content. Coagulation factors, including fibrinogen levels, VWF antigen and ristocetin cofactor assay, and clotting times (prothrombin time, international normalized ratio, and activated partial thromboplastin time) can indicate whether there are deficiencies or inhibitors of the coagulation cascade as an alternate (or concomitant) etiology for the patient's bleeding diathesis.

Formal evaluation of platelet function is performed by platelet aggregation assays in the clinical setting. These diagnostic tests are dependent on adequate platelet counts and are typically performed by impedance using whole blood aggregometry or light transmission aggregometry with platelet-rich plasma. Stimulation of platelets using a panel of agonists that typically includes ADP, arachidonic acid, epinephrine, collagen, ristocetin, and thrombin at low and high concentrations tests the ability of patient platelets to aggregate and secrete granules. Defects in one or both of these pathways can be measured and can suggest a platelet receptor defect or a storage pool disorder (**Table 1**). The traditional platelet aggregation assay is time-dependent and operator-dependent; automated platelet function screening tests include the PFA-100, which, although not specific for any disorder, can serve as a rapid screening test for platelet function.

Next generation sequencing for platelet disorders is becoming increasingly used, with commercial panels available for targeted gene sequencing of the causal genes for many inherited platelet disorders. At the time of this writing, turnaround time for most commercial panels is on the order of weeks, posing a major limitation for their use in clinical practice. Flow cytometry and electron microscopy of platelets can confirm a specific diagnosis by both qualitative and quantitative evaluation of platelet surface receptor and granule composition, although this is not routine in clinical practice.

Table 1
Platelet aggregation agonist response in inherited platelet disorders

Inherited Platelet Disorder	Ristocetin	ADP	Epinephrine	Arachidonic Acid	Collagen	Thrombin
Bernard-Soulier syndrome	Decreased	Normal	Normal	Normal	Normal	Normal
Glanzmann thrombasthenia	Normal	Decreased	Decreased	Decreased	Decreased	Decreased
Von Willebrand disease, type 2B (Montreal platelet syndrome)	Normal	Normal	Normal	Normal	Normal	Decreased
Signaling receptor defects	Variable response based on deficiency in specific agonist surface receptor					
Storage pool disorders	Decreased	Decreased	Decreased	Decreased	Decreased	Decreased
MYH9-associated disorders	Normal	Normal	Normal	Normal	Normal	Normal
Acquired platelet disorder (aspirin or NSAID use)	Normal	Decreased	Decreased	Decreased	Normal	Normal

The management of most congenital platelet disorders is supportive, with use of platelet transfusions and antifibrinolytic therapy with ε-aminocaproic acid or tranexamic acid to promote hemostasis. Desmopressin can induce release of endothelial VWF and promote platelet adhesion and aggregation in certain settings, though depending on the underlying defect may be of limited utility. Recombinant activated factor VII may be used urgently in the setting of uncontrolled bleeding. Unfortunately, recurrent platelet transfusions can increase the risk of platelet alloimmunization and refractoriness to subsequent platelet transfusions in patients. In these situations, and in severe thrombocytopenias related to defects in megakaryopoiesis and platelet production, allogeneic stem cell transplantation is often the only curative treatment modality. Gene therapy and replacement of the causal underlying genetic defect remains an area of active research investigation.

CONCLUSION

The diagnosis and recognition of inherited platelet disorders, although rare, is important in the evaluation and workup of bleeding. These disorders also highlight the clinical correlation between delayed hemostasis and the biology of platelet hematopoiesis and function. In clinical practice, awareness of an inherited platelet disorder is most significant to patients and providers and can allow for education and anticipatory guidance. Careful planning and consultation from a hematologist is needed in advance of any surgeries, pregnancies, or other procedures where bleeding is anticipated. Future advancements in the understanding of platelet biology and the mechanisms of congenital platelet disorders can lead to improvements in clinical diagnostics and management of patients with these rare diseases.

DISCLOSURES

F.D. Tsai: no conflicts of interest.

E.M. Battinelli: Sanofi, Consultant; American Society of Hematology, Speaker and Committee Member.

FUNDING SOURCES

This work was supported by National Institutes of Health, National Cancer Institute grant T32 CA009172 (F.D.T.).

REFERENCES

1. Broos K, Feys HB, De Meyer SF, et al. Platelets at work in primary hemostasis. Blood Rev 2011;25(4):155–67.
2. Lentaigne C, Freson K, Laffan MA, et al. Inherited platelet disorders: toward DNA-based diagnosis. Blood 2016;127(23):2814–23.
3. Savoia A, Kunishima S, De Rocco D, et al. Spectrum of the mutations in Bernard-Soulier syndrome. Hum Mutat 2014;35(9):1033–45.
4. Ali S, Shetty S, Ghosh K. A novel mutation in GP1BA gene leads to mono-allelic Bernard Soulier syndrome form of macrothrombocytopenia. Blood Coagul Fibrinolysis 2017;28(1):94–5.
5. Sivapalaratnam S, Westbury SK, Stephens JC, et al. Rare variants in GP1BB are responsible for autosomal dominant macrothrombocytopenia. Blood 2017; 129(4):520–4.
6. Noris P, Perrotta S, Bottega R, et al. Clinical and laboratory features of 103 patients from 42 Italian families with inherited thrombocytopenia derived from the monoallelic Ala156Val mutation of GPIbα (Bolzano mutation). Haematologica 2012;97(1):82–8.
7. Nurden AT, Fiore M, Nurden P, et al. Glanzmann thrombasthenia: a review of ITGA2B and ITGB3 defects with emphasis on variants, phenotypic variability, and mouse models. Blood 2011;118(23):5996–6005.
8. Manukjan G, Wiegering VA, Reindl T, et al. Novel variants in FERMT3 and RASGRP2-genetic linkage in Glanzmann-like bleeding disorders. Pediatr Blood Cancer 2020;67(2):e28078.
9. Kuijpers TW, van de Vijver E, Weterman MA, et al. LAD-1/variant syndrome is caused by mutations in FERMT3. Blood 2009;113(19):4740–6.
10. Robert P, Canault M, Farnarier C, et al. A novel leukocyte adhesion deficiency III variant: kindlin-3 deficiency results in integrin- and nonintegrin-related defects in different steps of leukocyte adhesion. J Immunol 2011;186(9):5273–83.
11. Lozano ML, Cook A, Bastida JM, et al. Novel mutations in RASGRP2, which encodes CalDAG-GEFI, abrogate Rap1 activation, causing platelet dysfunction. Blood 2016;128(9):1282–9.
12. Westbury SK, Canault M, Greene D, et al. Expanded repertoire of RASGRP2 variants responsible for platelet dysfunction and severe bleeding. Blood 2017; 130(8):1026–30.
13. Sevivas T, Bastida JM, Paul DS, et al. Identification of two novel mutations in RASGRP2 affecting platelet CalDAG-GEFI expression and function in patients with bleeding diathesis. Platelets 2018;29(2):192–5.
14. Jackson SC, Sinclair GD, Cloutier S, et al. The Montreal platelet syndrome kindred has type 2B von Willebrand disease with the VWF V1316M mutation. Blood 2009;113(14):3348–51.
15. Casari C, Berrou E, Lebret M, et al. von Willebrand factor mutation promotes thrombocytopathy by inhibiting integrin αIIbβ3. J Clin Invest 2013;123(12): 5071–81.
16. Offermanns S. Activation of platelet function through G protein-coupled receptors. Circ Res 2006;99(12):1293–304.

17. Rao AK, Jalagadugula G, Sun L. Inherited defects in platelet signaling mechanisms. Semin Thromb Hemost 2004;30(5):525–35.
18. Zwaal RF, Comfurius P, Bevers EM. Scott syndrome, a bleeding disorder caused by defective scrambling of membrane phospholipids. Biochim Biophys Acta 2004;1636(2–3):119–28.
19. Weiss HJ. Scott syndrome: a disorder of platelet coagulant activity. Semin Hematol 1994;31(4):312–9.
20. Chen Y, Yuan Y, Li W. Sorting machineries: how platelet-dense granules differ from α-granules. Biosci Rep 2018;38(5).
21. Ambrosio AL, Di Pietro SM. Storage pool diseases illuminate platelet dense granule biogenesis. Platelets 2017;28(2):138–46.
22. El-Chemaly S, Young LR. Hermansky-Pudlak Syndrome. Clin Chest Med 2016; 37(3):505–11.
23. Witkop CJ, Almadovar C, Piñeiro B, et al. Hermansky-Pudlak syndrome (HPS). An epidemiologic study. Ophthalmic Paediatr Genet 1990;11(3):245–50.
24. Buchanan GR, Handin RI. Platelet function in the Chediak-Higashi syndrome. Blood 1976;47(6):941–8.
25. Rendu F, Breton-Gorius J, Lebret M, et al. Evidence that abnormal platelet functions in human Chédiak-Higashi syndrome are the result of a lack of dense bodies. Am J Pathol 1983;111(3):307–14.
26. Introne W, Boissy RE, Gahl WA. Clinical, molecular, and cell biological aspects of Chediak-Higashi syndrome. Mol Genet Metab 1999;68(2):283–303.
27. Griscelli C, Durandy A, Guy-Grand D, et al. A syndrome associating partial albinism and immunodeficiency. Am J Med 1978;65(4):691–702.
28. Pastural E, Barrat FJ, Dufourcq-Lagelouse R, et al. Griscelli disease maps to chromosome 15q21 and is associated with mutations in the myosin-Va gene. Nat Genet 1997;16(3):289–92.
29. Ménasché G, Pastural E, Feldmann J, et al. Mutations in RAB27A cause Griscelli syndrome associated with haemophagocytic syndrome. Nat Genet 2000;25(2): 173–6.
30. Chen CH, Lo RW, Urban D, et al. α-granule biogenesis: from disease to discovery. Platelets 2017;28(2):147–54.
31. Blair P, Flaumenhaft R. Platelet alpha-granules: basic biology and clinical correlates. Blood Rev 2009;23(4):177–89.
32. Raccuglia G. Gray platelet syndrome. A variety of qualitative platelet disorder. Am J Med 1971;51(6):818–28.
33. Gunay-Aygun M, Zivony-Elboum Y, Gumruk F, et al. Gray platelet syndrome: natural history of a large patient cohort and locus assignment to chromosome 3p. Blood 2010;116(23):4990–5001.
34. Gunay-Aygun M, Falik-Zaccai TC, Vilboux T, et al. NBEAL2 is mutated in gray platelet syndrome and is required for biogenesis of platelet α-granules. Nat Genet 2011;43(8):732–4.
35. Monteferrario D, Bolar NA, Marneth AE, et al. A dominant-negative GFI1B mutation in the gray platelet syndrome. N Engl J Med 2014;370(3):245–53.
36. Tubman VN, Levine JE, Campagna DR, et al. X-linked gray platelet syndrome due to a GATA1 Arg216Gln mutation. Blood 2007;109(8):3297–9.
37. McKay H, Derome F, Haq MA, et al. Bleeding risks associated with inheritance of the Quebec platelet disorder. Blood 2004;104(1):159–65.
38. Kahr WH, Zheng S, Sheth PM, et al. Platelets from patients with the Quebec platelet disorder contain and secrete abnormal amounts of urokinase-type plasminogen activator. Blood 2001;98(2):257–65.

39. Liang M, Soomro A, Tasneem S, et al. Enhancer-gene rewiring in the pathogenesis of Quebec platelet disorder. Blood 2020;136(23):2679–90.

40. Chen Z, Naveiras O, Balduini A, et al. The May-Hegglin anomaly gene MYH9 is a negative regulator of platelet biogenesis modulated by the Rho-ROCK pathway. Blood 2007;110(1):171–9.

41. Kunishima S, Kobayashi R, Itoh TJ, et al. Mutation of the beta1-tubulin gene associated with congenital macrothrombocytopenia affecting microtubule assembly. Blood 2009;113(2):458–61.

42. Aguilar A, Pertuy F, Eckly A, et al. Importance of environmental stiffness for megakaryocyte differentiation and proplatelet formation. Blood 2016;128(16):2022–32.

43. Favier R, Raslova H. Progress in understanding the diagnosis and molecular genetics of macrothrombocytopenias. Br J Haematol 2015;170(5):626–39.

44. Donada A, Balayn N, Sliwa D, et al. Disrupted filamin A/α(IIb)β(3) interaction induces macrothrombocytopenia by increasing RhoA activity. Blood 2019; 133(16):1778–88.

45. Nurden P, Debili N, Coupry I, et al. Thrombocytopenia resulting from mutations in filamin A can be expressed as an isolated syndrome. Blood 2011;118(22): 5928–37.

46. Begonja AJ, Pluthero FG, Suphamungmee W, et al. FlnA binding to PACSIN2 F-BAR domain regulates membrane tubulation in megakaryocytes and platelets. Blood 2015;126(1):80–8.

47. Stritt S, Nurden P, Turro E, et al. A gain-of-function variant in DIAPH1 causes dominant macrothrombocytopenia and hearing loss. Blood 2016;127(23): 2903–14.

48. Burley K, Westbury SK, Mumford AD. TUBB1 variants and human platelet traits. Platelets 2018;29(2):209–11.

49. Nurden AT, Nurden P. Inherited thrombocytopenias: history, advances and perspectives. Haematologica 2020;105(8):2004–19.

50. Songdej N, Rao AK. Hematopoietic transcription factor mutations: important players in inherited platelet defects. Blood 2017;129(21):2873–81.

51. Favier R, Akshoomoff N, Mattson S, et al. Jacobsen syndrome: advances in our knowledge of phenotype and genotype. Am J Med Genet C Semin Med Genet 2015;169(3):239–50.

52. Vo KK, Jarocha DJ, Lyde RB, et al. FLI1 level during megakaryopoiesis affects thrombopoiesis and platelet biology. Blood 2017;129(26):3486–94.

53. Raslova H, Komura E, Le Couédic JP, et al. FLI1 monoallelic expression combined with its hemizygous loss underlies Paris-Trousseau/Jacobsen thrombopenia. J Clin Invest 2004;114(1):77–84.

54. Noetzli L, Lo RW, Lee-Sherick AB, et al. Germline mutations in ETV6 are associated with thrombocytopenia, red cell macrocytosis and predisposition to lymphoblastic leukemia. Nat Genet 2015;47(5):535–8.

55. Zhang MY, Churpek JE, Keel SB, et al. Germline ETV6 mutations in familial thrombocytopenia and hematologic malignancy. Nat Genet 2015;47(2):180–5.

56. Topka S, Vijai J, Walsh MF, et al. Germline ETV6 mutations confer susceptibility to acute lymphoblastic leukemia and thrombocytopenia. PLoS Genet 2015;11(6): e1005262.

57. Turro E, Greene D, Wijgaerts A, et al. A dominant gain-of-function mutation in universal tyrosine kinase SRC causes thrombocytopenia, myelofibrosis, bleeding, and bone pathologies. Sci Transl Med 2016;8(328):328ra30.

58. De Kock L, Thys C, Downes K, et al. De novo variant in tyrosine kinase SRC causes thrombocytopenia: case report of a second family. Platelets 2019;30(7): 931–4.

59. Barozzi S, Di Buduo CA, Marconi C, et al. Pathogenetic and clinical study of a patient with thrombocytopenia due to the p.E527K gain-of-function variant of SRC. Haematologica 2021;106(3):918–22.

60. Hamamy H, Makrythanasis P, Al-Allawi N, et al. Recessive thrombocytopenia likely due to a homozygous pathogenic variant in the FYB gene: case report. BMC Med Genet 2014;15:135.

61. Levin C, Koren A, Pretorius E, et al. Deleterious mutation in the FYB gene is associated with congenital autosomal recessive small-platelet thrombocytopenia. J Thromb Haemost 2015;13(7):1285–92.

62. Kahr WH, Pluthero FG, Elkadri A, et al. Loss of the Arp2/3 complex component ARPC1B causes platelet abnormalities and predisposes to inflammatory disease. Nat Commun 2017;8:14816.

63. Dowton SB, Beardsley D, Jamison D, et al. Studies of a familial platelet disorder. Blood 1985;65(3):557–63.

64. Ho CY, Otterud B, Legare RD, et al. Linkage of a familial platelet disorder with a propensity to develop myeloid malignancies to human chromosome 21q22.1-22.2. Blood 1996;87(12):5218–24.

65. Sood R, Kamikubo Y, Liu P. Role of RUNX1 in hematological malignancies. Blood 2017;129(15):2070–82.

66. Schlegelberger B, Heller PG. RUNX1 deficiency (familial platelet disorder with predisposition to myeloid leukemia, FPDMM). Semin Hematol 2017;54(2):75–80.

67. Pippucci T, Savoia A, Perrotta S, et al. Mutations in the 5' UTR of ANKRD26, the ankirin repeat domain 26 gene, cause an autosomal-dominant form of inherited thrombocytopenia, THC2. Am J Hum Genet 2011;88(1):115–20.

68. Noris P, Perrotta S, Seri M, et al. Mutations in ANKRD26 are responsible for a frequent form of inherited thrombocytopenia: analysis of 78 patients from 21 families. Blood 2011;117(24):6673–80.

69. Bluteau D, Balduini A, Balayn N, et al. Thrombocytopenia-associated mutations in the ANKRD26 regulatory region induce MAPK hyperactivation. J Clin Invest 2014; 124(2):580–91.

70. Ochs HD, Filipovich AH, Veys P, et al. Wiskott-Aldrich syndrome: diagnosis, clinical and laboratory manifestations, and treatment. Biol Blood Marrow Transplant 2009;15(1 Suppl):84–90.

71. Imai K, Morio T, Zhu Y, et al. Clinical course of patients with WASP gene mutations. Blood 2004;103(2):456–64.

72. Sereni L, Castiello MC, Di Silvestre D, et al. Lentiviral gene therapy corrects platelet phenotype and function in patients with Wiskott-Aldrich syndrome. J Allergy Clin Immunol 2019;144(3):825–38.

73. Ballmaier M, Germeshausen M, Schulze H, et al. c-mpl mutations are the cause of congenital amegakaryocytic thrombocytopenia. Blood 1 2001;97(1):139–46.

74. Ballmaier M, Schulze H, Strauss G, et al. Thrombopoietin in patients with congenital thrombocytopenia and absent radii: elevated serum levels, normal receptor expression, but defective reactivity to thrombopoietin. Blood 1997;90(2):612–9.

75. Letestu R, Vitrat N, Massé A, et al. Existence of a differentiation blockage at the stage of a megakaryocyte precursor in the thrombocytopenia and absent radii (TAR) syndrome. Blood 2000;95(5):1633–41.

76. Albers CA, Paul DS, Schulze H, et al. Compound inheritance of a low-frequency regulatory SNP and a rare null mutation in exon-junction complex subunit RBM8A causes TAR syndrome. Nat Genet 2012;44(4). 435-439, s1-s2.

77. Thompson AA, Woodruff K, Feig SA, et al. Congenital thrombocytopenia and radio-ulnar synostosis: a new familial syndrome. Br J Haematol 2001;113(4): 866–70.

78. Thompson AA, Nguyen LT. Amegakaryocytic thrombocytopenia and radio-ulnar synostosis are associated with HOXA11 mutation. Nat Genet 2000;26(4):397–8.

79. Niihori T, Ouchi-Uchiyama M, Sasahara Y, et al. Mutations in MECOM, encoding oncoprotein EVI1, cause radioulnar synostosis with amegakaryocytic thrombocytopenia. Am J Hum Genet 2015;97(6):848–54.

Von Willebrand Disease

Von Willebrand Disease
Current Status of Diagnosis and Management

Angela C. Weyand, MD[a], Veronica H. Flood, MD[b,c],*

KEYWORDS

- von Willebrand factor • von Willebrand disease • Bleeding • Coagulation factors

KEY POINTS

- VWD) is the most common inherited bleeding disorder.
- Multiple laboratory tests are needed for an accurate diagnosis of VWD.
- Treatment of patients with VWD includes desmopressin, antifibrinolytics, and von Willebrand factor concentrates.

INTRODUCTION

von Willebrand Disease (VWD), the most common inherited bleeding disorder, is defined by decreased activity of von Willebrand Factor (VWF) activity in the blood. This can be secondary to a quantitative or qualitative defect. VWF is a multimeric glycoprotein synthesized in endothelial cells and megakaryocytes and then stored within Weibel Palade bodies and alpha granules respectively. It is cleared by macrophages in the liver and spleen. Lack of VWF function, either through quantitative or qualitative defects, leads to a bleeding phenotype due to its critical role in primary and secondary hemostasis. Within primary hemostasis, VWF binds extracellular matrix proteins such as collagen, as well as platelets, through the glycoprotein Ib receptor. In secondary hemostasis, VWF acts as a chaperone to factor VIII (FVIII) to prevent premature clearance and degradation.

HISTORY

VWD was originally identified in 1926 by Dr Erik Adolf von Willebrand who described a familial pedigree of 58 individuals from 2 interrelated families spanning 4 generations. The proband was a 5-year-old girl who presented with recurrent severe mucosal bleeding and on testing demonstrated normal clotting time and clot retraction, but

[a] Department of Pediatrics, University of Michigan Medical School, 1150 W. Medical Center Dr, MSRB III, Room 8220E, Ann Arbor, MI 48109, USA; [b] Department of Pediatrics, Medical College of Wisconsin and Versiti Blood Research Institute, Milwaukee, WI, USA; [c] Comprehensive Center for Bleeding Disorders, 8739 Watertown Plank Road, PO Box 2178, Milwaukee, WI 53201-2178, USA
* Corresponding author.
E-mail address: vflood@mcw.edu

Hematol Oncol Clin N Am 35 (2021) 1085–1101
https://doi.org/10.1016/j.hoc.2021.07.004
0889-8588/21/© 2021 Elsevier Inc. All rights reserved.

hemonc.theclinics.com

marked prolongation of her bleeding time.[1,2] Within the pedigree, both male and female individuals were affected, and bleeding was severe, with multiple female family members, including the proband, dying secondary to mucosal bleeding. Diagnostic testing available in the early to mid-1900s was nonspecific, cumbersome, not reproducible, and time-consuming. Measurement of FVIII coagulation activity (FVIII:C) was first available in the mid-1900s and led to diagnostic confusion as deficiency was seen in classic hemophilia, as well as the condition later defined as VWD.[3,4] This led to the label of "pseudo-hemophilia," although others called the disorder "vascular hemophilia," as it was hypothesized that the prolonged bleeding time could be secondary to capillary defects.[5,6] Correction of the bleeding time defect with normal, as well as hemophilic plasma, confirmed that the defect lay outside of FVIII in the late 1950s[7] but it was not until the mid-1970s that VWF antigen testing was possible through immunoprecipitation.[8] A plethora of diagnostic assays have been developed, and development continues as currently available assays each have their own unique limitations.

PREVALENCE/INHERITANCE

The prevalence of VWD based on abnormal laboratory parameters alone is approximately 1 in 100, whereas the clinical prevalence, taking into consideration only those patients with bleeding symptoms, is likely closer to 1 in 1000.[9–11] VWD is inherited in an autosomal manner, so male and female individuals are affected equally. However, women are more likely to have symptomatic bleeding, given the additional hemostatic challenges of menstruation and childbirth.[12] Most commonly, VWD inheritance is autosomal dominant, but autosomal recessive inheritance is seen in type 3 and type 2N.[13] Type 1 VWD is the most common subtype, seen in 70% to 80% of patients with VWD. Type 2 is seen in approximately 20% of patients, and type 3 is rare, occurring in fewer than 5% of cases.[14]

SYMPTOMS

Mucocutaneous bleeding is common in patients with VWD, although symptoms are variable based on the subtype, level of VWF activity, age, and sex. The most commonly reported symptoms of VWD are outlined in **Table 1** [15,16] and should be specifically elucidated in the patient history. Particular attention should be paid to details of menses, as women may not recognize bleeding as abnormal, especially in the setting of a family history of similar bleeding.

Table 1	
Most commonly reported symptoms in patients with von Willebrand disease	
Symptom	**Proportion of Patients, %**
Heavy menstrual bleeding	75–100
Excessive bruising	62–81
Oropharyngeal bleeding	64
Epistaxis	56
Post dental procedure bleeding	26
Postsurgical bleeding	24
Excessive bleeding from wounds	24–58

In addition to mucocutaneous bleeding, patients with VWD may suffer from gastro-intestinal bleeding or joint bleeding. Recurrent gastrointestinal bleeding is a distinctive, difficult to treat, symptom of VWD that is often associated with angiodysplasia. It is more common in the elderly and in patients with type 2A and type 3 VWD. Joint bleeding is seen in 5% to 10% of patients with type 1 and type 2, and approximately 50% of patients with type 3.[17] Risk for joint bleeding is largely dependent on FVIII activity level and can lead to significant arthropathy.[18]

Standardized bleeding assessment tools (BATs) have been validated to help identify significant bleeding phenotypes,[19,20] although their utility is limited in younger patients who may not have encountered hemostatic challenges or in patients treated prophy-lactically. They also rely on cumulative scoring so that if a patient has previously had a lot of bleeding but is no longer having symptoms, their score will remain elevated. Last, they are easily saturable in that one episode of very severe bleeding within a subtype of bleeding will result in the same score as someone who has frequent episodes. Use of BATs is recommended when there is a low suspicion for VWD to help determine which patients require laboratory testing, but if a high suspicion for VWD exists, cur-rent guidelines suggest proceeding directly to laboratory testing.[21]

CLASSIFICATION

VWD can be due to a quantitative or qualitative deficiency of VWF and is subdivided into types based on the underlying defect. Types 1 and 3 are quantitative defects, with type 1 defined as a partial deficiency and type 3 resulting from an absolute deficiency of VWF. Type 1 includes type 1C, a subtype defined by increased clearance of VWF. Type 2 comprises qualitative defects and is further divided into multiple subtypes. Type 2A results from a defect in multimerization, whereas types 2B, 2N, and 2M are secondary to abnormal ligand binding: increased binding to platelet GPIb, defective binding to FVIII, and defective binding with normal multimers, respectively.

DIAGNOSIS

Testing for VWD should be performed only in patients with a personal or family history of bleeding. Once a personal or family history of bleeding has been established, lab-oratory testing is recommended. No single laboratory assay can definitively diagnose VWD. An algorithmic approach to diagnosis is outlined in **Fig. 1**. Diagnosis is further complicated by low penetrance, variable expressivity, laboratory variability, and the large number of modifiers affecting an individual's VWF level. Laboratories that use off-site processing are subject to many potential pre-analytical variables that affect VWF assays and can lead to falsely low levels and misdiagnosis of VWD.[22] VWF levels are influenced by genetic, environmental, hormonal, and pathologic processes. As an acute phase reactant, inflammatory processes cause elevation.[23,24] Similar increases are seen in pregnancy, aging, exercise, oral contraceptives, and exposure to cigarette smoke or air pollution.[25–30] As such, interpretation of VWF assays must be approached with caution and multiple evaluations are typically needed.

Screening assays, such as a complete blood count, activated partial thromboplastin time (aPTT) and prothrombin time, are likely to be normal in most patients with VWD and thus are of little utility. The aPTT may be prolonged in more severe cases and pa-tients with type 2B VWD may exhibit thrombocytopenia. Initial testing for VWD should include quantitative measurement with VWF antigen (VWF:Ag), a platelet binding assay such as the VWF-ristocetin cofactor assay (VWF:RCo) and FVIII:C. A functional assay is necessary, as antigen testing alone will miss some type 2 patients, and to classify types appropriately. Within these first-tier tests, clinical variability is significant

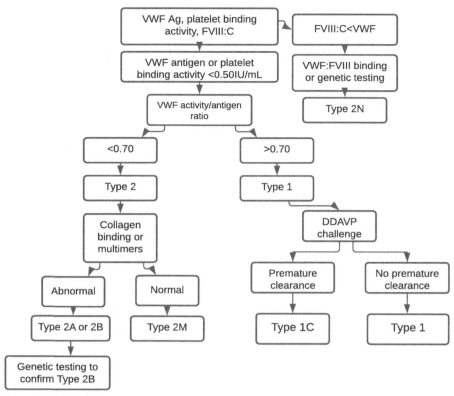

Fig. 1. An algorithmic approach to diagnosis.

at 30% for VWF:RCo and 20% for VWF:Ag,[31,32] although some observed differences in the VWF:Ag may be due to changes with age or stress.

The VWF:RCo assay is the most commonly used platelet binding assay and exploits the ristocetin-induced interaction between VWF and GPIb, which results in platelet agglutination. Although widely available, the VWF:RCo assay is limited by poor reproducibility, high coefficient of variation, low sensitivity at very low VWF levels, as well as falsely low VWF activity seen with certain benign sequence variations.[32,33] The p.D1472H variant has been seen in up to 67% of subjects with African ancestry and 20% of subjects with Caucasian backgrounds.[33] Given these limitations, other platelet binding assays have been developed. The VWF:GPIbM assay allows VWF to bind platelets spontaneously in vitro without the use of ristocetin by introduction 2 gain-of-function mutations into GPIbα.[34] Although results from VWF:RCo and VWF:GPIbM demonstrate a degree of correlation, GPIbM is more precise with a lower limit of detection of 2 IU/dL and a coefficient of variation of 5.6%[35] but is less readily available in many places. Neither assay is physiologic, as shear stress is not used to induce the VWF platelet interaction. The latest American Society of Hematology/International Society on Thrombosis and Haemostasis/National Hemophilia Foundation/World Federation of Hemophilia guidelines published earlier this year reviewed VWF:RCo, VWF:GPIbM, and VWF:GPIbR to reach a low certainty recommendation to use GPIbM. Although all 3 assays were judged to have comparable test accuracy in terms of sensitivity and specificity, the lower coefficient of variation, increased reproducibility, and lack of false positives due to benign sequence variations contributed to this recommendation.[21]

The platelet binding activity/VWF antigen ratio is used to differentiate between type 1 and type 2 VWD, with type 2 characterized by an activity/antigen ratio less than 0.7.[21] In addition to differentiating between type 1 and type 2 VWD, this ratio is essential in diagnosis, as some patients with type 2 VWD will have normal platelet binding activity and VWF antigen but an abnormal ratio. If the platelet binding activity/VWF antigen ratio is normal, consistent with a diagnosis of type 1 VWD, a desmopressin trial or the VWF propeptide (pp)/VWF antigen ratio can be used to evaluate for type 1C. Recent guidelines[21] recommend a desmopressin trial as the VWFpp/VWF:Ag ratio can be normal in the setting of rapid clearance.[36] If platelet binding activity/VWF:Ag ratio is <0.7, additional testing is necessary to identify the type 2 subtype. Multimer evaluation is performed using qualitative visual assessment and quantitative densitometric assessment by gel electrophoresis. Findings on multimer evaluation for VWD types are seen in **Fig. 2**. In addition to binding of FVIII and platelets, VWF also binds exposed collagen following vascular injury. VWF binds to multiple different collagen types and is dependent on high molecular weight (HMW) multimers. As binding to collagen types I and III is particularly reliant on HMW multimers, testing for this binding can serve as a surrogate for multimer analysis.[37] As such, this testing serves dual purposes of investigating for collagen defects, as well as evaluating multimer status. Of note, collagen binding defects have also been described in patients with type 1 VWD as well and are associated with a more severe phenotype.[38] Collagen binding or multimer analysis should be performed in patients suspected of having types 2A, 2B, and 2M. Abnormal VWF:CB and multimers is consistent with types 2A and 2B, whereas normal VWF:CB and multimers indicates a type 2M diagnosis.

Patients with type 2B VWD may have thrombocytopenia secondary to increased binding of VWF to platelets leading to premature clearance. Historically, ristocetin-induced platelet aggregation has been used to differentiate between types 2A and 2B. Using an aggregometer, various concentrations of ristocetin are added, and platelet aggregation measured. Aggregation at concentrations of 0.7 mg/mL or less are consistent with increased VWF binding to GPIb. Pathogenic variants that cause type 2B are found in exon 28, so targeted genetic testing can also be used. Patients with type 2N VWD can have normal or low normal levels of VWF in addition to low FVIII levels. The FVIII/VWF:Ag ratio can be used to help identify type 2N, as this group will have an FVIII/VWF:Ag ratio less than 0.6. As patients with hemophilia A will have a similar ratio, and FVIII is decreased, further testing should be performed to differentiate type 2N from hemophilia A. An enzyme-linked immunosorbent assay (ELISA) is available to evaluate VWF FVIII binding using an exogenous source of FVIII, as well as identify asymptomatic carriers.[39] Alternately, targeted genetic testing can be performed.[21] Given significant laboratory variability in type 2 diagnosis[40] and the importance of accurate subtyping, genetic testing has emerged as an adjunct for patients suspected of having type 2 VWD.

Genetic testing is being increasingly used in the diagnosis of VWD with increasing availability and decreasing costs. As with all testing, genetic testing is not without flaws. One drawback is the considerable variability seen in the VWF gene even within healthy cohorts.[41] For type 1, the most common subtype, there is weak correlation between sequence variants and disease.[42] A number of variants outside the VWF locus have also been implicated as modifiers of VWF levels including ABO blood group, CLEC4M, SCARA5, STXBP5, and UFM1.[43]

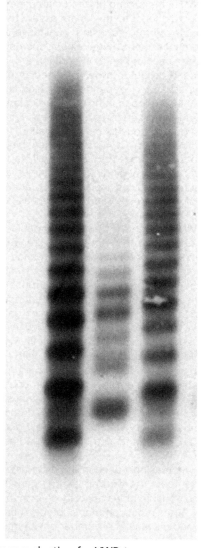

Fig. 2. Findings on multimer evaluation for VWD types.

CONTROVERSIES

One topic that has been the source of controversy is the laboratory threshold to meet diagnostic criteria for VWD. As previously discussed, approximately 1% of the population demonstrate low VWF levels on testing, but the prevalence of clinically relevant disease is likely much lower. As such, there is a good proportion of the population with low VWF levels without accompanying bleeding symptomatology. Conversely, mild bleeding symptoms are also commonly reported in healthy populations.[44] Patients with VWF levels less than 30 IU/dL are more likely to have VWF coding mutations and autosomal dominant family inheritance[45] compared with those with levels of 30 to 50 IU/dL. Given the differences in these 2 groups, some have advocated that patients with VWF levels between 30 and 50 IU/dL be labeled as having low VWF, a modest risk factor for bleeding, rather than diagnosed with a disease. The most recent guidelines strongly recommend a diagnosis of VWD in patients with a bleeding history and levels less than 50 IU/dL. Of note, these guidelines referenced data demonstrating similar bleeding across the range of VWF levels,[42,46] as well as data demonstrating significant bleeding in most patients with VWF levels between 30 and 50 IU/dL.[47] Clinician judgment remains an important consideration, and patients with modest decrease in VWF level may require evaluation for additional bleeding disorders such as platelet function defects that could contribute to the bleeding phenotype.

Another area of dispute relates to the increase in VWF levels that is seen with normal aging.[48] Given this, patients, especially those with modestly low levels at diagnosis, may have levels in the normal range at older ages. Observational studies have shown that this normalization occurs in approximately 43% of patients.[21] It is not known whether this normalization of levels translates to decreased risk for bleeding. One study examining bleeding symptoms in patients with type 1 VWD found that patients older than 65 years experienced as much bleeding as those 18 to 65 years of age.[49] As such, the normal increase in levels seen with age may not correlate with normalization of bleeding. The recent VWD guidelines addressed the question of whether patients whose levels normalize with age should still carry a diagnosis of VWD and recommended reconsidering the diagnosis, rather than removing it.[21] Interestingly, type 2 VWD patients may see an increase in antigen levels but still have dysfunctional protein and report increased bleeding with age.[49] Conversely, one study that evaluated VWF levels in young children before tonsillectomy found decreased levels to be relatively common and not predictive of bleeding risk,[50] suggesting bleeding history may be as important as the absolute VWF level.

TREATMENT

Treatment of VWD centers around replacing the deficient or defective VWF. For patients with a history of frequent severe bleeding, long-term prophylaxis with VWF replacement is recommended.[51] A randomized controlled trial comparing prophylaxis to on-demand treatment found extended time to first bleed, reduced bleeding episode risk, and decreased epistaxis with prophylaxis.[52] Observational trials have similarly demonstrated reduced bleeding episodes, hospitalizations, and heavy menstrual bleeding with prophylaxis.[53–61] Current products available for VWF replacement include plasma derived and recombinant products, as well as products with and without FVIII. Commercially available products and dosing recommendations can be found in **Table 2**. When using combined VWF/FVIII products, it is important to note that once infused, the half-life of FVIII is longer than that of VWF. In addition to the exogenously infused FVIII, the infused VWF will stabilize endogenous FVIII, which can lead to accumulation. Elevated FVIII levels are a risk factor for the development of

Table 2
Currently approved von Willebrand factor (VWF) concentrates in the United States

Product	Type	VWF RCo:VWF Ag Ratio	VWF RCo:FVIII Ratio	Mean Half-Life, h
Alphanate	Plasma derived	0.47 ± 0.1	1.33 ± 0.26	17.9 ± 9.6
Humate	Plasma derived	0.59 ± 0.1	2.45 ± 0.3	~ 12.2
Vonvendi	Recombinant	1.16 ± 0.25	No FVIII	21.9 ± 8.36
Wilate	Plasma derived	Not available	1.0	19.6 ± 6.9

venous thromboembolism (VTE)[62] and cases of VTE have been described in patients with VWD with elevated FVIII secondary to treatment.[63] Replacement products with VWF alone may be preferable in patients with other risk factors for thrombosis.[64] For patients with VWD and associated low FVIII levels, replacement products with VWF alone require an FVIII priming dose or sufficient time for endogenous levels to rise. Compiled recommendations for surgical prophylaxis can be found in **Table 3**.

In many patients with type 1 and type 2 VWD, desmopressin, a synthetic analog of vasopressin, can be used to increase VWF levels without VWF replacement, and is the most widely used therapy in VWD.[65] Desmopressin stimulates release of endogenous VWF and FVIII from endothelial cells, leading to a transient increase in levels. It is available in intravenous (IV), subcutaneous (SC), and intranasal (IN) preparations. Recommended IV and SC dosing is 0.3 μg/kg of body weight (up to 20 μg), and IN dosing is 150 μg (1 spray) in patients less than 50 kg or 300 μg (2 sprays) in patients greater than 50 kg. SC and IV formulations increase VWF and FVIII levels 2 to 4 times baseline within 30 to 60 minutes of administration[66] and can be repeated every 12 to 24 hours. Tachyphylaxis (reduced response to successive doses) occurs after 2 to 3 days. The intranasal formulation has variable absorption and results in a more modest increase in levels. Not all patients with VWD will respond to desmopressin. Given its mechanism of action, it requires a pool of endogenous VWF and therefore is not effective or recommended in type 3 VWD. Desmopressin is generally contraindicated in patients with type 2B VWD, as increasing defective VWF can lead to increased binding of VWF and platelets, worsening thrombocytopenia. Although many patients with type 2A and 2M VWD may have improvement of minor symptoms with desmopressin, VWF levels typically do not have a sufficient rise with desmopressin to allow its use for surgery or major bleeds. Patients with type 1C VWD are characterized by premature clearance of desmopressin, so identification of these patients is imperative, as they are likely to demonstrate an initial response followed by a drop to baseline within 2 to 4 hours.

A desmopressin trial is recommended to diagnose type 1C and before use in patients with type 1 and levels less than 30 IU/dL.[21,51] Most type 1 patients are responsive to desmopressin.[67,68] In adults, patients with levels greater than 30 IU/dL typically respond to desmopressin,[51] so may not require a trial before use. There is no consensus for how a desmopressin trial is conducted, but FVIII and VWF levels are commonly assessed at baseline, 1 hour post infusion, and 4 hours post infusion. Response has also been defined variably with a recent proposal to define it as an increase of at least 2 times baseline VWF activity level and sustained increase of FVIII and VWF above 50 IU/dL for at least 4 hours.[69] As this level is inadequate for some procedures, desmopressin-responsive patients may at times require VWF concentrate. Adverse effects of desmopressin are typically mild (tachycardia, flushing, headache) but occur frequently. Due to its antidiuretic effect, there is a risk of hyponatremia and fluid overload. As this risk is greatest in the youngest children, its use is not recommended in children younger than 2 years.[51] For all others, fluid restriction and

Table 3
Recommendations for surgical prophylaxis

	Preoperative VWF:RCo	Preoperative FVIII:C	Postoperative VWF:RCo	Postoperative FVIII:C
Major surgery				
Nichols et al,[91] 2008	>100	>100	≥50 for 7–10 d	≥50 for 7–10 d
Laffan et al,[80] 2014	>100	>100		>50
Castman et al,[92] 2013	80–100	80–100	80–100 for 36h, >50 for 5–10 d	
Windyga et al,[93] 2016	>50	>80–100	>30 for days 1–14	>50 for days 1–7, >30 for days 8–14
Connell et al,[51] 2021			≥50 for at least 3 d	≥50 for at least 3 d
Minor surgery				
Nichols et al,[91] 2008	>30, preferably >50	>30, preferably >50	>30, preferably >50 for 3–5 d	>30, preferably >50, for 3–5 d
Laffan et al,[80] 2013	>50	>50		
Castman et al,[92] 2013		>30		>30 2–4 d
Windyga et al,[93] 2016	>50	>80–100	>30 for 3–5 d	>50 for 3–5 d
Connell et al,[51] 2021	≥50 + TXA or TXA alone in type 1 VWD patient with levels >30, mild bleeding phenotype and minor mucosal procedure			

Abbreviations: C, coagulation; FVIII, factor VIII; RCo, ristocetin cofactor; TXA, tranexamic acid; VWD, von Willebrand disease; VWF, von Willebrand factor.
Data from Refs[51,80,91–93]

electrolyte monitoring when repeated doses are given is recommended. Desmopressin is not recommended for use in patients with active cardiovascular disease, seizure disorders, women with preeclampsia, and patients with type 1C VWD in situations that require sustained response.[51]

Supportive treatments, such as hormonal treatments and antifibrinolytics, are commonly used in patients with VWD depending on the type of bleeding. Tranexamic acid and ε-aminocaproic acid are antifibrinolytics that act by blocking plasminogen binding sites to prevent fibrin degradation. Due to high fibrinolytic activity in mucosal tissue, antifibrinolytics are particularly helpful for mucosal bleeding.[70] Antifibrinolytics also play a role in the treatment of heavy menstrual bleeding. Tranexamic acid (TXA) has been shown to decrease menstrual blood loss (MBL) by 50%[71] and in a randomized controlled crossover trial demonstrated greater efficacy than desmopressin in reducing MBL in patients with VWD.[72] Due to their low cost and favorable side-effect profile, they are often used as an adjunct in other settings. Antifibrinolytics can be given systemically, via IV or oral formulations, or topically. They should not be used in patients with urinary tract bleeding, as this can lead to clotting and ureteral obstruction.[73]

Given the high rate of HMB in women with VWD, hormonal treatments are also commonly used. In women not desiring pregnancy, combined hormonal contraceptives (CHC) and the levonorgestrel intrauterine device (IUD) have shown benefit in decreasing MBL. CHCs lead to nonovulatory bleeding and decreased bleeding during the placebo week when taken cyclically and greatly reduce days of bleeding when taken continuously.[74] The IUD decreases MBL by increasing capillary thrombosis and suppressing endometrium and spiral arteriole growth. A systematic review found that in comparison with TXA and CHC, IUDs decreased MBL by both objective and subjective measures.[75] In patients with HMB desiring pregnancy, TXA is recommended.[51] Women with HMB also should be assessed and treated for iron deficiency and iron deficiency anemia.

In addition to heavy menstrual bleeding, women with VWD are at risk for bleeding associated with pregnancy and delivery. In the case of pregnancy in a patient with VWD, a multidisciplinary approach should be used with input from hematology, pediatric hematology, obstetrics, and anesthesiology. During pregnancy, women undergo physiologic changes to tip the balance of hemostasis toward a procoagulant state to prepare for delivery.[76] Many changes occur, including an increase in VWF and FVIII, which both peak shortly after birth and return to normal by 12 weeks postpartum.[77] In patients with type 1 VWD, VWF and FVIII levels increase over the course of pregnancy, particularly during the third trimester to 2 to 3 times their baseline level at delivery.[78] Unfortunately, not all women, even those with mild disease, mount this physiologic response. In type 2 patients, VWF:Ag and FVIII levels may increase but function remains abnormal. In patients with type 3 VWD, VWF and FVIII remain low throughout the pregnancy. Given the variable increase in FVIII and VWF during pregnancy, VWF testing, including functional activity, antigen, and FVIII, should be done between 30 and 34 weeks' gestation.[79] Prior guidelines suggest treating with desmopressin or factor concentrate for functional VWF levels less than 50 IU/dL.[80] However, this has been debated in recent years given data on type 1 VWD with postpartum hemorrhage (PPH) despite normalization of endogenous VWF and FVIII levels.[81] Furthermore, in another study, PPH was seen in 50% of patients with VWD treated with VWF concentrate targeting levels greater than 100 IU/dL, suggesting that women with VWD may need higher levels in the postpartum setting.[82]

Women with VWD who desire or require neuraxial anesthesia during delivery should receive VWF concentrate to achieve VWF levels of 50 to 150 IU/dL,[51] although higher levels may be required to prevent PPH. TXA has also been shown to decrease the risk of PPH in women with and without bleeding disorders.[83,84] TXA is recommended post-partum for women with type 1 VWD, as well as possibly type 2 and type 3 VWD[51] with recommendations to continue for 7 to 15 days depending on bleeding risk.[85]

COMPLICATIONS

A rare complication of VWD is the development of alloantibodies. It is estimated that 5% to 10% of patients with type 3 VWD will develop antibodies following VWF factor concentrate administration.[86] Patients with partial or complete gene deletions are at highest risk.[87] The development of inhibitors renders treatment with VWF concentrate ineffective. Recombinant FVIII products have shown to be effective for procedural hemostasis, but prophylactic use is limited given the incredibly short half-life in the absence of VWF.[88] Bypassing agents such as recombinant factor VIIa are also used,[89] and recent reports demonstrate efficacy with emicizumab, a bispecific antibody FVIII mimetic.[90]

Another challenging situation is the development of comorbidities that require the use of antiplatelet or anticoagulant therapy. Despite bleeding risk, patients with VWD requiring antiplatelet or anticoagulation therapy should receive this treatment. Patients at severe risk for bleeding may require specific VWF replacement to mitigate this risk.[51] Careful clinical monitoring is indicated with regular reassessment of risk.

SUMMARY

Optimal treatment for patients with VWD requires suspicion of the diagnosis because specific testing is required. Understanding the available laboratory tests is also important to determine if a patient has VWD, and if so, what type of VWD is present, as that will help determine appropriate treatment. Accurate treatment of VWD ameliorates bleeding symptoms and improves quality of life for patients with VWD.

CLINICS CARE POINTS

- Patients with significant history of mucosal bleeding merit evaluation for VWD.
- Accurate diagnosis requires evaluation of VWF antigen, as well as platelet binding activity to determine if a patient has a quantitative (type 1 or type 3) or a qualitative (type 2) defect in VWF.
- Although most patients with type 1 VWD respond well to desmopressin, there are patients with clearance defects and a short VWF half-life who require treatment with VWF concentrate.

ACKNOWLEDGMENT

The authors would like to acknowledge NIH funding (HL126810 to VHF).

DISCLOSURE STATEMENT

The authors have nothing to disclose.

REFERENCES

1. von Willebrand AE. Hereditar pseudohemofili. Finska Lakarsall-skapetes Handl 1926;67:7–112.

2. Lassila R, Lindberg O. Erik von Willebrand. Haemophilia 2013;19(5):643–7.

3. Biggs R, Eveling J, Richards G. The assay of antihaemophilic-globulin activity. Br J Haematol 1955;1(1):20–34.

4. Hardisty RM, MacPherson JC. A one-stage factor VIII (antihaemophilic globulin) assay and its use on venous and capillary plasma. Thromb Diath Haemorrh 1962; 7:215–28.

5. Alexander B, Goldstein R. Dual hemostatic defect in pseudohemophilia. J Clin Invest 1953;32:551.

6. Erlandson M, Fort E, Lee RE, et al. Vascular hemophilia; a familial hemorrhagic disease in males and females characterized by combined antihemophilic globulin deficiency and vascular abnormality. Pediatrics 1956;18(3):347–61.

7. Cornu P, Larrieu MJ, Caen J, et al. Transfusion studies in von Willebrand's disease: effect on bleeding time and factor VIII. Br J Haematol 1963;9:189–202.

8. Zimmerman TS, Hoyer LW, Dickson L, et al. Determina- tion of the von Wille-brand's disease antigen (factor VIII-related antigen) in plasma by quantitative immunoelectrophoresis. J Lab Clin Med 1975;86(1):152–9.

9. Rodeghiero F, Castaman G, Dini E. Epidemiological investigation of the preva-lence of von Willebrandos disease. Blood 1987;69:454–9.

10. Werner EJ, Broxson EH, Tucker EL, et al. Prevalence of von Willebrand disease in children: a multiethnic study. J Pediatr 1993;123:893–8.

11. Bowman M, Hopman WM, Rapson D, et al. The prevalence of symptomatic von Willebrand disease in primary care practice. J Thromb Haemost 2010;8(1):213–6.

12. De Wee EM, Knol HM, Mauser-Bunschoten EP, et al. Gynaecological and obstet-ric bleeding in moderate and severe von Willebrand disease. Thromb Haemost 2011;106:885–92.

13. Itzhar-Baikian N, Boisseau P, Joly B, et al. Updated overview on von Willebrand disease: focus on the interest of genotyping. Expert Rev Hematol 2019;12(12): 1023–36.

14. Leebeek FW, Eikenboom JC. Von Willebrand's Disease. N Engl J Med 2016; 375(21):2067–80.

15. James PD, Notley C, Hegadorn C, et al. The mutational spectrum of type 1 von Willebrand disease: results from a Canadian cohort study. Blood 2007;109(1): 145–54.

16. Sanders YV, Fijnvandraat K, Boender J, et al, WiN Study Group. Bleeding spec-trum in children with moderate or severe von Willebrand disease: Relevance of pediatric-specific bleeding. Am J Hematol 2015;90(12):1142–8.

17. van Galen KP, Sanders YV, Vojinovic U, et al, WiN Study Group. Joint bleeds in von Willebrand disease patients have significant impact on quality of life and joint integrity: a cross-sectional study. Haemophilia 2015;21(03):e185–92.

18. van Galen KPM, Mauser-Bunschoten EP, Leebeek FWG. Hemophilic arthropathy in patients with von Willebrand disease. Blood Rev 2012;26:261–6.

19. Rodeghiero F, Tosetto A, Abshire T, et al. ISTH/SSC joint VWF and Perinatal/Pedi-atric Hemostasis Subcommittees Working Group. ISTH/SSC bleeding assess-ment tool: a standardized questionnaire and a proposal for a new bleeding score for inherited bleeding disorders. J Thromb Haemost 2010;8(9):2063–5.

20. Bowman ML, James PD. Bleeding scores for the diagnosis of von Willebrand dis-ease. Semin Thromb Hemost 2017;43(5):530–9.

21. James PD, Connell NT, Ameer B, et al. ASH ISTH NHF WFH Guidelines on the diagnosis of von Willebrand disease. Blood Adv 2021;5(1):280–300.

22. Jaffray J, Staber JM, Malvar J, et al. Laboratory misdiagnosis of von Willebrand disease in post-menarchal females: a multi-center study. Am J Hematol 2020; 95(9):1022–9.

23. Pottinger B, Read R, Paleolog E, et al. von Willebrand factor is an acute phase reactant in man. Thromb Res 1989;53:387–94.

24. Kremer Hovinga JA, Zeerleder S, Kessler P, et al. ADAMTS-13, von Willebrand factor and related parameters in severe sepsis and septic shock. J Thromb Haemost 2007;5:2284–90.

25. Castaman G. Changes of von Willebrand factor during pregnancy in women with and without von Willebrand disease. Mediterr J Hematol Infect Dis 2013;5: e2013052.

26. Ribeiro J, Almeida-Dias A, Ascens~ao A, et al. Hemostatic response to acute physical exercise in healthy adolescents. J Sci Med Sport 2007;10:164–9.

27. Timm A, Fahrenkrug J, Jørgensen HL, et al. Diurnal variation of von Willebrand factor in plasma: the Bispebjerg study of diurnal variations. Eur J Haematol 2014;93:48–53.

28. Al-Awadhi AM, Alfadhli SM, Mustafa NY, et al. Effects of cigarette smoking on hematological parameters and von Willebrand factor functional activity levels in asymptomatic male and female Arab smokers. Med Princ Pract 2008;17:149–53.

29. Yuan Z, Chen Y, Zhang Y, et al. Changes of plasma vWF level in response to the improvement of air quality: an observation of 114 healthy young adults. Ann Hematol 2013;92:543–8.

30. Kouides PA. Aspects of the laboratory identification of von Willebrand disease in women. Semin Thromb Hemost 2006;32:480–4.

31. Hayes TE, Brandt JT, Chandler WL, et al. External peer review quality assurance testing in von Willebrand disease: the recent experience of the United States College of American Pathologists proficiency testing program. Semin Thromb Hemost 2006;32:499–504.

32. Kitchen S, Jennings I, Woods TA, et al. Laboratory tests for measurement of von Willebrand factor show poor agreement among different centers: results from the United Kingdom national external quality assessment scheme for blood coagulation. Semin Thromb Hemost 2006;32:492–8.

33. Flood VH, Gill JC, Morateck PA, et al. Common VWF exon 28 polymorphisms in African Americans affecting the VWF activity assay by ristocetin cofactor. Blood 2010;116:280–6.

34. Patzke J, Budde U, Huber A, et al. Performance evaluation and multicentre study of a von Willebrand factor activity assay based on GPIb binding in the absence of ristocetin. Blood Coagul Fibrinolysis 2014;25(8):860–70.

35. Graf L, Moffat KA, Carlino SA, et al. Evaluation of an automated method for measuring von Willebrand factor activity in clinical samples without ristocetin. Int J Lab Hematol 2014;36(3):341–51.

36. Haberichter SL, Castaman G, Budde U, et al. Identification of type 1 von Willebrand disease patients with reduced von Willebrand factor survival by assay of the VWF propeptide in the European study: molecular and clinical markers for the diagnosis and management of type 1 VWD (MCMDM-1VWD). Blood 2008; 111(10):4979–85.

37. Favaloro EJ. An update on the von Willebrand factor collagen binding assay: 21 years of age and beyond adolescence but not yet a mature adult. Semin Thromb Hemost 2007;33(8):727–44.

38. Flood VH, Schlauderaff AC, Haberichter SL, et al, Zimmerman Program Investigators. Crucial role for the VWF A1 domain in binding to type IV collagen. Blood 2015;125(14):2297–304.
39. Casonato A, Pontara E, Zerbinati P, et al. A. Girolami. The evaluation of factor VIII binding activity of von Willebrand factor by means of an ELISA method: significance and practical implications. Am J Clin Pathol 1998;109:347–52.
40. DiGiandomenico S, Christopherson PA, Haberichter SL, et al, Zimmerman Program Investigators. Laboratory variability in the diagnosis of type 2 VWD variants. J Thromb Haemost 2021;19(1):131–8.
41. Bellissimo DB, Christopherson PA, Flood VH, et al. VWF mutations and new sequence variations identified in healthy controls are more frequent in the African-American population. Blood 2012;119:2135–40.
42. Flood VH, Christopherson PA, Gill JC, et al. Clinical and laboratory variability in a cohort of patients diagnosed with type 1 VWD in the United States. Blood 2016; 127(20):2481–8.
43. Sharma R, Flood VH. Advances in the diagnosis and treatment of Von Willebrand disease. Blood 2017;130(22):2386–91.
44. Sadler JE. Low von Willebrand factor: sometimes a risk factor and sometimes a disease. Hematol Am Soc Hematol Educ Program 2009;106–12.
45. O'Donnell JS, Low VWF. insights into pathogenesis, diagnosis, and clinical management. Blood Adv 2020;4(13):3191–9.
46. Lavin M, Aguila S, Schneppenheim S, et al. Novel insights into the clinical phenotype and pathophysiology underlying low VWF levels. Blood 2017;130(21): 2344–53.
47. Bucciarelli P, Siboni SM, Stufano F, et al. Predictors of von Willebrand disease diagnosis in individuals with borderline von Willebrand factor plasma levels. J Thromb Haemost 2015;13(2):228–36.
48. Rydz N, Grabell J, Lillicrap D, et al. Changes in von Willebrand factor level and von Willebrand activity with age in type 1 von Willebrand disease. Haemo- philia 2015;21:636–41.
49. Sanders YV, Giezenaar MA, Laros-van Gorkom BAP, et al. Von Willebrand disease and aging: an evolving phenotype. J Thromb Haemost 2014;12:1066–75.
50. Gill JC, Conley SF, Johnson VP, et al. Low VWF levels in children and lack of association with bleeding in children undergoing tonsillectomy. Blood Adv 2020; 4(1):100–5.
51. Connell NT, Flood VH, Brignardello-Peterson R, et al. ASH ISTH NHF WFH guidelines on the management of von Willebrand disease. Blood Adv 2021;5(1): 301–25.
52. Peyvandi F, Castaman G, Gresele P, et al. A phase III study comparing secondary long-term prophylaxis versus on-demand treatment with vWF/FVIII concentrates in severe inherited von Willebrand disease. Blood Transfus 2019;17(5):391–8.
53. Berntorp E, Petrini P. Long-term prophylaxis in von Willebrand disease. Blood Coagul Fibrinolysis 2005;16(suppl 1):S23–6.
54. Berntorp E, Windyga J, European Wilate Study Group. Treatment and prevention of acute bleedings in von Willebrand disease–efficacy and safety of Wilate, a new generation von Willebrand factor/factor VIII concentrate. Haemophilia 2009;15(1): 122–30.
55. Borel-Derlon A, Federici AB, Roussel-Robert V, et al. Treatment of severe von Willebrand disease with a high-purity von Willebrand factor concentrate (Wilfactin): a prospective study of 50 patients. J Thromb Haemost 2007;5(6):1115–24.

56. Federici AB, Barillari G, Zanon E, et al. Efficacy and safety of highly purified, doubly virus-inactivated VWF/FVIII concentrates in inherited von Willebrand's disease: results of an Italian cohort study on 120 patients characterized by bleeding severity score. Haemophilia 2010;16(1):101–10.
57. Holm E, Abshire TC, Bowen J, et al. Changes in bleeding patterns in von Willebrand disease after institution of long-term replacement therapy: results from the von Willebrand Disease Prophylaxis Network. Blood Coagul Fibrinolysis 2015;26(4):383–8.
58. Abshire T, Cox-Gill J, Kempton CL, et al. Prophylaxis escalation in severe von Willebrand disease: a prospective study from the von Willebrand Disease Prophylaxis Network. J Thromb Haemost 2015;13(9):1585–9.
59. Abshire TC, Federici AB, Alvarez MT, et al, VWD PN. Prophylaxis in severe forms of von Willebrand's disease: results from the von Willebrand Disease Prophylaxis Network (VWD PN). Haemophilia 2013;19(1):76–81.
60. Holm E, Carlsson KS, Lövdahl S, et al. Bleeding-related hospitalization in patients with von Willebrand disease and the impact of prophylaxis: Results from national registers in Sweden compared with normal controls and participants in the von Willebrand Disease Prophylaxis Network. Haemophilia 2018;24(4):628–33.
61. Federici AB. Highly purified VWF/FVIII concentrates in the treatment and prophylaxis of von Willebrand disease: the PRO. WILL study. Haemophilia 2007; 13(suppl 5):15–24.
62. Tsai AW, Cushman M, Rosamond WD, et al. Coagulation factors, inflammation markers, and venous thromboembolism: the longitudinal investigation of thromboembolism etiology (LITE). Am J Med 2002;113(8):636–42.
63. Makris M, Colvin B, Gupta V, et al. Venous thrombosis following the use of intermediate purity FVIII concentrate to treat patients with von Willebrand's disease. Thromb Haemost 2002;88(3):387–8.
64. Weyand AC, Jesudas R, Pipe SW. Advantage of recombinant von Willebrand factor for peri-operative management in paediatric acquired von Willebrand syndrome. Haemophilia 2018;24(3):e120–1.
65. Heijdra JM, Cnossen MH, Leebeek FWG. Current and emerging options for the management of inherited von Willebrand disease. Drugs 2017;77(14):1531–47.
66. Castaman G. How I treat von Willebrand disease. Thromb Res 2020;196:618–25.
67. Ben-Ami T, Revel-Vilk S. The use of DDAVP in children with bleeding disorders. Pediatr Blood Cancer 2013;60(Suppl 1):S41–3.
68. Federici AB. The use of desmopressin in von Willebrand disease: the experience of the first 30 years (1977-2007). Haemophilia 2007;14(suppl 1):5–14.
69. Connell NT, James PD, Brignardello-Petersen R, et al. von Willebrand disease: proposing definitions for future research. Blood Adv 2021;5(2):565–9.
70. Sindet-Pedersen S. Haemostasis in oral surgery—the possible pathogenetic implications of oral fibrinolysis on bleeding. Experimental and clinical studies of the haemostatic balance in the oral cavity, with particular reference to patients with acquired and congenital defects of the coagulation system Review. Dan Med Bull 1991;38(6):427–43.
71. Bryant-Smith AC, Lethaby A, Farquhar C, et al. Antifibrinolytics for heavy menstrual bleeding. Cochrane Database Syst Rev 2018;4(4):CD000249.
72. Kouides PA, Byams VR, Philipp CS, et al. Multisite management study of menorrhagia with abnormal laboratory haemostasis: a prospective crossover study of intranasal desmopressin and oral tranexamic acid. Br J Haematol 2009;145(2): 212–20.

73. Koo JR, Lee YK, Kim YS, et al. Acute renal cortical necrosis caused by an anti-fibrinolytic drug (tranexamic acid). Nephrol Dial Transplant 1999;14(3):750–2.
74. Kwiecien M, Edelman A, Nichols MD, et al. Bleeding patterns and patient accept-ability of standard or continuous dosing regimens of a low-dose oral contracep-tive: a randomized trial. Contraception 2003;67(1):9–13.
75. Bofill Rodriguez M, Lethaby A, Jordan V. Progestogen-releasing intrauterine sys-tems for heavy menstrual bleeding. Cochrane Database Syst Rev 2020;6(6): CD002126.
76. Brenner B. Haemostatic changes in pregnancy. Thromb Res 2004;114(5–6): 409–14.
77. Nowak-Göttl U, Limperger V, Kenet G, et al. Developmental hemostasis: a life-span from neonates and pregnancy to the young and elderly adult in a European white population. Blood Cells Mol Dis 2017;67:2–13.
78. Sánchez-Luceros A, Meschengieser SS, Marchese C, et al. Factor VIII and von Willebrand factor changes during normal pregnancy and puerperium. Blood Coagul Fibrinolysis 2003;14(7):647–51.
79. Leebeek FWG, Duvekot J, Kruip MJHA. How I manage pregnancy in carriers of hemophilia and patients with von Willebrand disease. Blood 2020;136(19): 2143–50.
80. Laffan MA, Lester W, O'Donnell JS, et al. The diagnosis and management of von Willebrand disease: a United Kingdom Haemophilia Centre Doctors Organization guideline approved by the British Committee for Standards in Haematology. Br J Haematol 2014;167(4):453–65.
81. Punt MC, Waning ML, Mauser-Bunschoten EP, et al. Maternal and neonatal bleeding complications in relation to peripartum management in women with Von Willebrand disease: a systematic review. Blood Rev 2020;39:100633.
82. Stoof SC, van Steenbergen HW, Zwagemaker A, et al. Primary postpartum hae-morrhage in women with von Willebrand disease or carriership of haemophilia despite specialised care: a retrospective survey. Haemophilia 2015;21(4): 505–12.
83. WOMAN Trial Collaborators. Effect of early tranexamic acid administration on mortality, hysterectomy, and other morbidities in women with post-partum hae-morrhage (WOMAN): an international, randomised, double-blind, placebo-controlled trial. Lancet 2017;389(10084):2105–16.
84. Kouides PA. Antifibrinolytic therapy for preventing VWD-related postpartum hem-orrhage: indications and limitations. Blood Adv 2017;1(11):699–702.
85. Castaman G, James PD. Pregnancy and delivery in women with von Willebrand disease. Eur J Haematol 2019;103(2):73–9.
86. James PD, Lillicrap D, Mannucci PM. Alloantibodies in von Willebrand disease. Blood 2013;122(5):636–40.
87. Federici AB. Clinical and molecular markers of inherited von Willebrand disease type 3: are deletions of the VWF gene associated with alloantibodies to VWF? J Thromb Haemost 2008;6(10):1726–8.
88. Pergantou H, Xafaki P, Adamtziki E, et al. The challenging management of a child with type 3 von Willebrand disease and antibodies to von Willebrand factor. Hae-mophilia 2012;18(3):e66–7.
89. Franchini M, Mannucci PM. Alloantibodies in von Willebrand disease. Semin Thromb Hemost 2018;44(6):590–4.
90. Weyand AC, Flood VH, Shavit JA, et al. Efficacy of emicizumab in a pediatric pa-tient with type 3 von Willebrand disease and alloantibodies. Blood Adv 2019; 3(18):2748–50.

91. Nichols WL, Hultin MB, James AH, et al. von Willebrand disease (VWD): evidence-based diagnosis and management guidelines, the National Heart, Lung, and Blood Institute (NHLBI) Expert Panel report (USA). Haemophilia 2008;14(2):171–232.
92. Castaman G, Goodeve A, Eikenboom J, European Group on von Willebrand Disease. Principles of care for the diagnosis and treatment of von Willebrand disease. Haematologica 2013;98(5):667–74.
93. Windyga J, Dolan G, Altisent C, et al, EHTSB. Practical aspects of factor concentrate use in patients with von Willebrand disease undergoing invasive procedures: a European survey. Haemophilia 2016;22(5):739–51.

Acquired von Willebrand Syndrome

Arielle L. Langer, MD, MPH, Nathan T. Connell, MD, MPH*

KEYWORDS

- Acquired von Willebrand • Essential thrombocythemia
- Waldenström macroglobulinemia • Mechanical circulatory support • Aortic stenosis
- Shear forces • Mucocutaneous bleeding
- Gastrointestinal arteriovenous malformations

KEY POINTS

- Diagnosis should be suspected in patients with mucocutaneous bleeding and a predisposing condition.
- Myeloproliferative neoplasms, plasma cell dyscrasias (PCD), and cardiovascular disease, including aortic stenosis and mechanical circulatory support, are the most common causes.
- Treatment should be focused on the underlying disease when possible.

INTRODUCTION

Although von Willebrand factor (VWF) was initially characterized in the setting of an inherited bleeding disorder, individuals may also develop a deficiency of VWF during their lifetime, termed acquired von Willebrand syndrome (AVWS). AVWS may arise from a heterogenous group of mechanisms, but share a common set of features (**Table 1**).

In 1958, Dr Edward Heyde first reported a link between aortic and gastrointestinal (GI) bleeding.[1] Nearly 30 years later, this association was proven[2] and the presence of low VWF was noted in certain cardiac surgery patients with bleeding,[3] but it was several more years before AVWS was proposed as the link between these observations.[4] Since that time AVWS has gained recognition and been shown to be associated with several cardiac, hematologic, and autoimmune disorders.

EPIDEMIOLOGY

The exact frequency of AVWS is difficult to ascertain, because it is underdiagnosed and increasing in incidence and prevalence.[5,6] Underdiagnosis is likely driven by attribution of bleeding to comorbidities and lack of consideration of this rare diagnosis,

Division of Hematology, Brigham and Women's Hospital, 75 Francis Street, Boston, MA 02115, USA
* Corresponding author.
E-mail address: ntconnell@bwh.harvard.edu

Hematol Oncol Clin N Am 35 (2021) 1103–1116
https://doi.org/10.1016/j.hoc.2021.07.005
hemonc.theclinics.com

Table 1
Causes of Acquired von Willebrand Syndrome

Causes	Examples and Prevalence of AVWS in Each Condition if Available
Shear forces	Aortic stenosis (Heyde syndrome): prevalence 67%–92% by laboratory criteria; bleeding seen in 21%[25] Congenital heart defects: prevalence 20.8% by laboratory criteria[33] Other structural defects: mitral regurgitation, hypertrophic obstructive cardiomyopathy Extracorporeal membrane oxygenation: prevalence up to 100% by laboratory criteria; bleeding seen in 68.8%–94.4%[11,17] Ventricular assist device: prevalence up to 100% by laboratory criteria; bleeding seen in 19%–59%[38,39,43,45,46] Short-term microaxial pumps: prevalence 95.2% by laboratory criteria[47]
Myeloproliferative neoplasms	Essential thrombocythemia: prevalence 20%–70% by laboratory criteria; bleeding in <50% of laboratory diagnoses[7,54–56] Polycythemia vera: prevalence 12%–30% by laboratory criteria; bleeding in <50% of laboratory diagnoses[7,54,57] Chronic myelogenous leukemia
Lymphoproliferative disorders	Monoclonal gammopathy of undetermined significance Waldenström macroglobulinemia: prevalence 14% by laboratory criteria[9] Multiple myeloma AL amyloidosis Chronic lymphocytic leukemia Other lymphomas
Autoimmune disorders	Systemic lupus erythematosus Rheumatoid arthritis Graft-versus-host disease Isolated von Willebrand factor inhibitor
Other	Wilms tumor Other solid tumors Hypothyroidism Medications: griseofulvin, ciprofloxacin, valproic acid, hydroxyethyl starch

and the existence subclinical AVWS.[7–13] However, better recognition is not solely responsible for increasing diagnosis, because the true prevalence is rising, caused by the aging of the population leading to a great prevalence of age-related conditions, such as monoclonal gammopathy of undetermined significance (MGUS)[14] and aortic stenosis[15,16] and caused by the use of mechanical circulatory support, such as ventricular assist devices (VADs) and extracorporeal membrane oxygenation (ECMO).[6,10,11,17–21] We group the etiologies as arising from shear forces, myeloproliferative neoplasms (MPNs), plasma cell dyscrasias (PCD) and other lymphoproliferative disorders, autoimmune disorders, and other conditions.

Shear Forces

Mechanical shearing leads to AVWS by activation of high-molecular-weight (HMW) VWF multimers and subsequent removal from circulation.[11,22–24] There is also evidence of increased cleavage by ADAMTS13 (a disintegrin and metalloproteinase with a thrombospondin type 1 motif, member 13) and mechanical destruction of VWF.[19] Increased shear forces can arise from structural heart disease, prototypically aortic stenosis, or from the use of mechanical circulatory support. The rate of AVWS is 67% to 92% of patients with severe aortic stenosis, although only a smaller proportion of patients (21%) have bleeding manifestation.[25] The valve gradient has been shown to be correlated with the degree of disturbance in multimer patterns and likelihood of bleeding.[26,27] The causal link was proven by the observations that correction of aortic stenosis is associated with resolution of bleeding and normalization of VWF multimers.[25,28]

In addition to aortic stenosis, other structural defects that have been associated with AVWS include mitral regurgitation, hypertrophic obstructive cardiomyopathy, and congenital heart defects, and are well documented to correct with repair of the structural defect.[29–37] The rates for AVWS in congenital heart defects vary widely by defect: one study of 192 patients seen in an adult congenital heart defect clinic found an overall AVWS prevalence of 20.8% with a range of 9.4% in patients with less complex defects and 38.6% in patients with the most complex defects in the cohort.[33] Another series that focused on congenital heart defects with a stenotic component found AVWS rates of 50% in those with a significant gradient (mean, 80; range, 52–130 mm Hg), as compared with no children with a gradient less than 20 mm Hg,[34] further emphasizing the role of shear forces.

Mechanical circulatory support is increasing in prevalence and increasingly recognized to cause AVWS. Venovenous and venoarterial ECMO have been shown to cause AVWS.[10,11,17–19,21] One series of 18 venovenous ECMO patients found laboratory evidence of ECMO in all 18 patients with 17 of the 18 showing clinical signs of bleeding,[11] whereas another series of 32 venoarterial ECMO patients found laboratory evidence in 31 and bleeding in 22 patients, respectively.[17] Similarly, laboratory evidence of AVWS in VAD patients was seen in all 102 patients in one series.[38] Bleeding represents the most common complication of VAD implantation and is impacted by, although not exclusively caused by, AVWS with rates varying from 19% to 59% depending on the study.[23,39–46] Newer devices with lower shear stress seem to have lower rates of AVWS.[19] AVWS can also occur with short-term microaxial pumps with laboratory evidence in 20 of 21 patients in one series.[47–49] AVWS caused by mechanical circulatory support typically resolves with decannulation or device removal.[11,40,50]

Myeloproliferative Neoplasms

The markedly increased platelet counts that are see with MPNs are thought to underly the association with AVWS in most cases. This is most commonly reported with essential thrombocythemia but also in patients with polycythemia vera and chronic myelogenous leukemia when the platelet count is concurrently elevated.[7,51,52] The likelihood of AVWS is correlated with the degree of thrombocytosis and is unusual without a platelet count of greater than $1000 \times 10^9/L$, although cases have been reported at lower platelet counts, because the mechanism is adsorption on the surface of excessive platelets, which preferentially impacts HMW multimers.[7,8,53,54] Estimates for AVWS are 20% to 70% in essential thrombocythemia and 12% to 30% in polycythemia vera by laboratory criteria, but clinically significant bleeding is much less common, at 4% to 7% in some studies and affecting fewer than half of those with a laboratory-based diagnosis.[7,54–57]

Plasma Cell Dyscrasias and Other Lymphoproliferative Disorders

AVWS has been associated with PCD through adsorption by paraproteins and acquisition of an autoantibody to VWF, which is termed a VWF inhibitor.[9,51,58–61] PCD includes AL amyloidosis, MGUS, multiple myeloma, and Waldenström macroglobulinemia. In a series of 72 patients with Waldenström macroglobulinemia, 10 patients (14%) met laboratory criteria for AVWS.[9] Rates for multiple myeloma and MGUS are not well characterized, but occur with IgG and IgM subtypes.[5,51,58] Likewise, AVWS is a rare complication of AL amyloidosis, but can occur with kappa and lambda subtypes.[60,61] Although the proportion of PCD patients with AVWS is likely low, because of the prevalence of these disorders, PCD accounts for a large proportion of identified cases, as high as 48% in a registry of 211 patients.[5] Rarely other lymphoproliferative disorders including chronic lymphocytic leukemia and other lymphomas have been associated with AVWS.[5,51]

Autoimmune Disorders

Autoimmune AVWS can occur in the setting of PCD. Autoimmune AVWS has also been documented to occur in the setting of systemic autoimmune disorders. This is most commonly in association with systemic lupus erythematosus,[62–69] but has also been reported with rheumatoid arthritis[70,71] and graft-versus-host disease.[72] AVWS as an isolated inhibitor without evidence of other autoimmunity or systemic disease has also been reported.[73,74]

Other Etiologies

Rare cases of AVWS have also been reported with several other conditions. Solid tumors, including most notably Wilms tumor, have been associated with rare cases.[5,51,75] Hypothyroidism has been associated with AVWS with a normal multimer pattern and resolution with administration of L-thyroxine, implying diminished synthesis can occur in this setting.[76–78] Rarely, AVWS has been associated with medications including griseofulvin,[79] ciprofloxacin,[80] valproic acid,[81] and hydroxyethyl starch.[82–84] Drug-induced AVWS can involve loss across all multimer forms (eg, hydroxyethyl starch, valproic acid) or be limited to HMW multimers (eg, ciprofloxacin).

EVALUATION
Diagnosing Acquired von Willebrand Syndrome

Patients with suspected AVWS based on either clinical symptoms or a predisposing condition should have VWF testing (**Table 2**). This testing should include VWF antigen levels and ristocetin cofactor assay or equivalent test of VWF platelet binding activity. Normal results for VWF antigen levels and VWF ristocetin cofactor assay effectively

Table 2
Laboratory Profile of Acquired von Willebrand Syndromes

Laboratory Parameter	Type 1 AVWS	Type 2A AVWS
VWF:Ag	Low	Low, normal, or high
VWF:RCo	Low, in proportion to VWF:Ag	Low, out of proportion to VWF:Ag
VWF multimer analysis	Normal distribution	HMW multimer diminished or absent
Testing to distinguish from inherited VWD	Genetic testing or VWFpp[a]	Genetic testing, elevation of VWF:Ag if present, VWFpp

Abbreviations: HMW, high molecular weight; VWD, von Willebrand disease; VWF:Ag, von Willebrand factor antigen levels; VWF:RCo, von Willebrand factor ristocetin cofactor assay; VWFpp, von Willebrand factor propeptide.
[a] Rare this may misidentify type 1C VWD as acquired and hypothyroidism-associated type 1 AVWS as congenital.

rule out AVWS. If either is abnormal, VMF multimer analysis can distinguish the AVWS subtype. A global decrease with a normal multimer pattern is equivalent to type 1 von Willebrand disease (VWD) (or type 3 if sufficiently severe), whereas selective loss of HMW multimers is analogous to type 2A VWD. When suspicion is high or diagnosis is time sensitive, it may be appropriate to send multimer testing with the initial evaluation. Multimer analysis is helpful not only in establishing the diagnosis, but also in selection of therapy (discussed later).

Distinguishing Acquired von Willebrand Syndrome From von Willebrand Factor

Clinical history is often able to distinguish AVWS from inherited VWD by the abrupt onset of bleeding symptoms or the novel presence of a predisposing condition (eg, essential thrombocythemia diagnosis or VAD placement). As such, a careful bleeding history is of vital importance to rule out an occult bleeding history, particularly that of heavy menstrual bleeding, which patients may not recognize as excessive because of lack of context for comparison or may be hesitant to disclose because of historical stigmatization of menses.[85]

When clinical history is insufficient, additional testing is of use.[13] Few patients have prior VWF testing for comparison, but this would differentiate AVWS from VWD if available. Normal or elevated VWF propeptide can distinguish AVWS caused by increased clearance, which represents most AVWS, from VWD.[86,87] However, one should be cautious relying on propeptide testing without understanding the clinical context as would result in cases of AVWS caused by reduced production (eg, hypothyroidism)[76–78] being mislabeled as type 1 VWD and cases of type 1C VWD being mislabeled as AVWS. Gene sequencing to assess for mutations, inversions, and deletes associated with VWD can provide clarity when clinical context or other laboratory testing is insufficient to make the determination.

For patients in whom an autoimmune mechanism is suspected, testing directly for an inhibitor can confirm the diagnosis and help tailor therapy.

Assessing for Underlying Conditions

Most AVWS is associated with a predisposing condition[5] and that is often apparent before the diagnosis of AVWS or readily apparent from the patient's history. For those patients without a known cause, a complete blood count should be reviewed for evidence of MPN or cytopenias suggestive of an underlying disorder. A serum protein electrophoresis and free light chain ratio may be useful to screen for PCD. Patients with inhibitors should be screened for systemic lupus erythematosus and hematologic malignancies including PCD. Cardiac auscultation may reveal previously unappreciated aortic stenosis. Testing for more obscure causes should be clinically driven.

CLINICAL OUTCOMES

The clinical presentation of AVWS can vary widely in severity. Many cases with clear laboratory evidence suggesting AVWS may be clinically silent.[7,9,17,25,56,57] Cases with clinical manifestations can present with mucocutaneous bleeding including petechiae, bruising, gum bleeding, epistaxis, heavy menstrual bleeding and GI bleeding.[51] GI bleeding is the most common site of life-threatening bleeding, although bleeding can been seen at any site including airways, pericardium, pleural space, and peritoneum.[6,10,39,51]

Subtypes of AVWS where HMW multimers are preferentially impacted are most likely to manifest bleeding, because these multimers are the most hemostatically active. Furthermore, in patients with a loss of HMW multimers, GI bleeding may be driven not only because of the hemostatic defect, but also by the development of arteriovenous malformations (AVMs). The propensity of patients with AVWS with loss of HMW multimers to form AVMs is thought to be central to the original observation linking aortic stenosis to GI bleeding in Heyde syndrome.[1,2,4] VWF, and HMW multimers in particular, play a role in regulation of angiogenesis, which may be tissue specific and account for GI AVMs.[88–90] As such, recurrent GI AVMs should prompt clinical consideration of underlying VWD or AVWS.

THERAPEUTIC OPTIONS

The most effective long-term therapy for AVWS usually addresses the predisposing condition. This has been shown to be effective in most causes,[25,28–31,35,37,50,54,55,57] but this approach is not always feasible and does not address acute bleeding (**Table 3**).

Acute Bleeding

Desmopressin, which is routinely used for type 1 VWD, generally performs poorly as a rescue therapy for bleeding with great heterogeneity across AVWS causes.[5,6,51,58,77,91] Response rates to desmopressin were 10% for cardiovascular causes, 21% for MPNs, 33% for autoimmune conditions, and 44% for PCD and lymphomas.[5] Mechanistically, low response rates are not surprising, because a transient release of endothelial stores

Table 3 Treatments for Acquired von Willebrand Syndrome		
Therapy	**Dosing**	**Considerations**
VWF concentrates	Initial: 40–60 U/kg Maintenance: 40–50 U/kg daily	Fast onset; short duration of effect
Desmopressin	0.3 µg/kg, max 20 µg	Fast onset; poor efficacy; short duration of effect
Intravenous immunoglobulins	Initial: 1 g/kg q d × 2 d Maintenance: 1 g/kg q 3 wk	Fast onset; significant volume load
Antifibrinolytics		
Tranexamic acid ε-Aminocaproic acid	1–1.3 g IV or PO q 8 h IV: 4–5 g loading dose followed by 1 g/h continuous infusion or PO: 50–100 mg/kg q 6 h	Adjunctive therapy for bleeding refractory to other therapies
B-cell-directed therapy		
Rituximab	Initial: 375 mg/m² weekly × 4 doses Maintenance (optional): 375 mg/m² q 90 d or with relapse	Slow onset; may provide long treatment-free interval
Bortezomib	1.3 mg/m² (+dexamethasone 40 mg) on D1, 4, 8, and 11 of 21-d cycles × 6 cycles	Slow onset; response in rituximab refractory patient
Antiangiogenic therapy		
Thalidomide	50 mg PO BID	Slow onset; prothrombotic
Octreotide	Short acting: 50 µg SC BID; Depo: 20 mg SC monthly	Slow onset; gastrointestinal, cardiovascular and endocrinologic side effects

Abbreviations: IV, intravenous; SC, subcutaneous.

of VWF does not address the rapid clearance of VWF underlying most AVWS. The use of VWF concentrates may be more successful than desmopressin, although data are limited, with a response rate of 40% across underlying causes.[5,10,20,58,92] Intravenous immunoglobulin (IVIG) has shown success in MGUS, lymphoproliferative disorders, autoimmune conditions, and solid tumors with response rates ranging from 37% to 100%.[5,58,59,92,93] It is physiologically plausible that immune clearance of VWF is halted by IVIG administration, which may explain its success in this particular subset of AVWS. This theory is bolstered by the observation that high success rates in IgG MGUS are not found with IgM MGUS, where adsorption rather than targeted clearance may be underlying.[9,58,94] Plasmapheresis is effective for IgM MGUS or Waldenström macroglobulinemia.[58,59] Antifibrinolytics, such as tranexamic acid and ε-aminocaproic acid, have also been suggested to ameliorate acute bleeding, but data are lacking.[6] One series reported the successful use of recombinant activated factor VII to halt bleeding in AVWS.[95]

Prophylaxis Against Future Bleeding

Correction of the underlying condition is the optimal approach, but this may be impossible in many circumstances. For conditions discussed previously that are responsive to IVIG, including IgG MGUS, other PCD, and autoimmune causes, repeat administration every 3 weeks may provide long-term control.[93,96] If an inhibitor is identified or suspected, B-cell therapy, such as the anti-CD20 monoclonal antibody rituximab, has generated long-term responses[64,96–100]; however, rituximab failure in MGUS-associated AVWS has been reported.[101] There is a case report of successful treatment of MGUS-associated AVWS with bortezomib.[102]

Patients for whom the previously mentioned therapies are insufficient or are not expected to be effective and have developed recurrent GI AVMs may be considered for antiangiogenic therapies. This is particularly relevant to patients with VADs, because there is no expectation of resolving AVWS without heart transplantation. Factor replacement alone is likely to be insufficient, because accelerated clearance makes it difficult to maintain VWF levels. For the combination of GI bleeding and VAD, the antiangiogenic medications octreotide and thalidomide have reduced GI bleeding.[103–109]

CLINICS CARE POINTS

- Recurrent GI AVMs should prompt consideration of underlying AVWS.
- Diagnostic testing should include VWF multimer analysis to identify the decrease in HMW multimers.
- Multimer pattern, history, and clinical context can usually distinguish AVWS from VWD; however, genetic testing may be needed to distinguish AVWS from type 2A VWD.
- Treatment should target the underlying condition when possible (eg, correction of aortic stenosis, removal of mechanical circulatory support, treatment of an MPN or PCD).
- Desmopressin performs poorly in AVWS, especially when caused by underlying cardiovascular causes.
- VWF concentrates may be effective to treat acute bleeding episodes.
- IVIG is effective for rapid and long-term correction of AVWS in lymphoproliferative and autoimmune conditions.
- Patients with recurrent AVMs despite treatment may benefit from antiangiogenic therapies.

DISCLOSURE

The authors have no conflicts of interest to disclose.

REFERENCES

1. Heyde EC. Gastrointestinal bleeding in aortic stenosis. N Engl J Med 1958; 259(4):196.
2. Greenstein RJ, McElhinney AJ, Reuben D, et al. Colonic vascular ectasias and aortic stenosis: coincidence or causal relationship? Am J Surg 1986;151(3): 347–51.
3. Salzman EW, Weinstein MJ, Weintraub RM, et al. Treatment with desmopressin acetate to reduce blood loss after cardiac surgery. N Engl J Med 1986;314(22): 1402–6.
4. Warkentin TE, Moore JC, Morgan DG. Aortic stenosis and bleeding gastrointestinal angiodysplasia: is acquired von Willebrand's disease the link? Lancet Lond Engl 1992;340(8810):35–7.
5. Federici AB, Rand JH, Bucciarelli P, et al. Acquired von Willebrand syndrome: data from an international registry. Thromb Haemost 2000;84(2):345–9.
6. Tiede A, Rand JH, Budde U, et al. How I treat the acquired von Willebrand syndrome. Blood 2011;117(25):6777–85.
7. Fabris F, Casonato A, Grazia del Ben M, et al. Abnormalities of von Willebrand factor in myeloproliferative disease: a relationship with bleeding diathesis. Br J Haematol 1986;63(1):75–83.
8. Awada H, Voso MT, Guglielmelli P, et al. Essential thrombocythemia and acquired von Willebrand syndrome: the shadowlands between thrombosis and bleeding. Cancers 2020;12(7):1746.
9. Hivert B, Caron C, Petit S, et al. Clinical and prognostic implications of low or high level of von Willebrand factor in patients with Waldenstrom macroglobulinemia. Blood 2012;120(16):3214–21.
10. Mazzeffi M, Bathula A, Tabatabai A, et al. Von Willebrand factor concentrate administration for acquired von Willebrand syndrome-related bleeding during adult extracorporeal membrane oxygenation. J Cardiothorac Vasc Anesth 2020;35(3):882–7.
11. Kalbhenn J, Schmidt R, Nakamura L, et al. Early diagnosis of acquired von Willebrand syndrome (AVWS) is elementary for clinical practice in patients treated with ECMO therapy. J Atheroscler Thromb 2015;22(3):265–71.
12. Budde U, Bergmann F, Michiels JJ. Acquired von Willebrand syndrome: experience from 2 years in a single laboratory compared with data from the literature and an international registry. Semin Thromb Hemost 2002;28(2):227–38.
13. Tiede A, Priesack J, Werwitzke S, et al. Diagnostic workup of patients with acquired von Willebrand syndrome: a retrospective single-centre cohort study. J Thromb Haemost JTH 2008;6(4):569–76.
14. Kyle RA, Therneau TM, Rajkumar SV, et al. Prevalence of monoclonal gammopathy of undetermined significance. N Engl J Med 2006;354(13):1362–9.
15. Eveborn GW, Schirmer H, Heggelund G, et al. The evolving epidemiology of valvular aortic stenosis. The Tromsø study. Heart Br Card Soc 2013;99(6): 396–400.
16. Stewart BF, Siscovick D, Lind BK, et al. Clinical factors associated with calcific aortic valve disease. Cardiovascular Health Study. J Am Coll Cardiol 1997;29(3): 630–4.

17. Heilmann C, Geisen U, Beyersdorf F, et al. Acquired von Willebrand syndrome in patients with extracorporeal life support (ECLS). Intensive Care Med 2012; 38(1):62–8.
18. Malfertheiner MV, Pimenta LP, Bahr V von, et al. Acquired von Willebrand syndrome in respiratory extracorporeal life support: a systematic review of the literature. Crit Care Resusc J Australas Acad Crit Care Med 2017;19(Suppl 1): 45–52.
19. Schlagenhauf A, Kalbhenn J, Geisen U, et al. Acquired von Willebrand syndrome and platelet function defects during extracorporeal life support (mechanical circulatory support). Hamostaseologie 2020;40(2):221–5.
20. Rauch A, Susen S, Zieger B. Acquired von Willebrand syndrome in patients with ventricular assist device. Front Med 2019;6:7.
21. Tamura T, Horiuchi H, Obayashi Y, et al. Acquired von Willebrand syndrome in patients treated with veno-arterial extracorporeal membrane oxygenation. Cardiovasc Interv Ther 2019;34(4):358–63.
22. Tauber H, Ott H, Streif W, et al. Extracorporeal membrane oxygenation induces short-term loss of high-molecular-weight von Willebrand factor multimers. Anesth Analg 2015;120(4):730–6.
23. Geisen U, Heilmann C, Beyersdorf F, et al. Non-surgical bleeding in patients with ventricular assist devices could be explained by acquired von Willebrand disease. Eur J Cardio-thorac Surg 2008;33(4):679–84.
24. Brophy TM, Ward SE, McGimsey TR, et al. Plasmin cleaves von Willebrand factor at K1491-R1492 in the A1-A2 linker region in a shear- and glycan-dependent manner in vitro. Arterioscler Thromb Vasc Biol 2017;37(5):845–55.
25. Vincentelli A, Susen S, Le Tourneau T, et al. Acquired von Willebrand syndrome in aortic stenosis. N Engl J Med 2003;349(4):343–9.
26. Blackshear JL, Wysokinska EM, Safford RE, et al. Indexes of von Willebrand factor as biomarkers of aortic stenosis severity (from the Biomarkers of Aortic Stenosis Severity [BASS] study). Am J Cardiol 2013;111(3):374–81.
27. Natorska J, Bykowska K, Hlawaty M, et al. Increased thrombin generation and platelet activation are associated with deficiency in high molecular weight multimers of von Willebrand factor in patients with moderate-to-severe aortic stenosis. Heart Br Card Soc 2011;97(24):2023–8.
28. Yamashita K, Yagi H, Hayakawa M, et al. Rapid restoration of thrombus formation and high-molecular-weight von Willebrand factor multimers in patients with severe aortic stenosis after valve replacement. J Atheroscler Thromb 2016; 23(10):1150–8.
29. Horiuchi H, Doman T, Kokame K, et al. Acquired von Willebrand syndrome associated with cardiovascular diseases. J Atheroscler Thromb 2019;26(4):303–14.
30. Blackshear JL, Schaff HV, Ommen SR, et al. Hypertrophic obstructive cardiomyopathy, bleeding history, and acquired von Willebrand syndrome: response to septal myectomy. Mayo Clin Proc 2011;86(3):219–24.
31. Wake M, Takahashi N, Yoshitomi H, et al. A case of hypertrophic obstructive cardiomyopathy and acquired von Willebrand syndrome: response to medical therapy. J Echocardiogr 2014;12(3):112–4.
32. Onimoe G, Grooms L, Perdue K, et al. Acquired von Willebrand syndrome in congenital heart disease: does it promote an increased bleeding risk? Br J Haematol 2011;155(5):622–4.
33. Waldow HC, Westhoff-Bleck M, Widera C, et al. Acquired von Willebrand syndrome in adult patients with congenital heart disease. Int J Cardiol 2014; 176(3):739–45.

34. Loeffelbein F, Funk D, Nakamura L, et al. Shear-stress induced acquired von Willebrand syndrome in children with congenital heart disease. Interact Cardiovasc Thorac Surg 2014;19(6):926–32.

35. Blackshear JL, Wysokinska EM, Safford RE, et al. Shear stress-associated acquired von Willebrand syndrome in patients with mitral regurgitation. J Thromb Haemost JTH 2014;12(12):1966–74.

36. Wan S-H, Liang JJ, Vaidya R, et al. Acquired Von Willebrand syndrome secondary to mitral and aortic regurgitation. Can J Cardiol 2014;30(9):1108.e9-10.

37. Kasai M, Osako M, Inaba Y, et al. Acquired von Willebrand syndrome secondary to mitral and aortic regurgitation. J Card Surg 2020;35(9):2396–8.

38. Meyer AL, Malehsa D, Budde U, et al. Acquired von Willebrand syndrome in patients with a centrifugal or axial continuous flow left ventricular assist device. JACC Heart Fail 2014;2(2):141–5.

39. Uriel N, Pak S-W, Jorde UP, et al. Acquired von Willebrand syndrome after continuous-flow mechanical device support contributes to a high prevalence of bleeding during long-term support and at the time of transplantation. J Am Coll Cardiol 2010;56(15):1207–13.

40. Meyer AL, Malehsa D, Bara C, et al. Acquired von Willebrand syndrome in patients with an axial flow left ventricular assist device. Circ Heart Fail 2010;3(6):675–81.

41. Muslem R, Caliskan K, Leebeek FWG. Acquired coagulopathy in patients with left ventricular assist devices. J Thromb Haemost 2018;16(3):429–40.

42. Kirklin JK, Naftel DC, Pagani FD, et al. Seventh INTERMACS annual report: 15,000 patients and counting. J Heart Lung Transpl 2015;34(12):1495–504.

43. Lahpor J, Khaghani A, Hetzer R, et al. European results with a continuous-flow ventricular assist device for advanced heart-failure patients. Eur J Cardio-thorac Surg 2010;37(2):357–61.

44. Starling RC, Naka Y, Boyle AJ, et al. Results of the post-U.S. Food and Drug Administration-approval study with a continuous flow left ventricular assist device as a bridge to heart transplantation: a prospective study using the INTERMACS (Interagency Registry for Mechanically Assisted Circulatory Support). J Am Coll Cardiol 2011;57(19):1890–8.

45. Draper KV, Huang RJ, Gerson LB. GI bleeding in patients with continuous-flow left ventricular assist devices: a systematic review and meta-analysis. Gastrointest Endosc 2014;80(3):435–46.e1.

46. Demirozu ZT, Radovancevic R, Hochman LF, et al. Arteriovenous malformation and gastrointestinal bleeding in patients with the HeartMate II left ventricular assist device. J Heart Lung Transplant 2011;30(8):849–53.

47. Flierl U, Tongers J, Berliner D, et al. Acquired von Willebrand syndrome in cardiogenic shock patients on mechanical circulatory microaxial pump support. PLoS One 2017;12(8):e0183193.

48. Goldfarb M, Czer LS, Lam LD, et al. High molecular weight von Willebrand factor multimer loss and bleeding in patients with short-term mechanical circulatory support devices: a case series. J Extra Corpor Technol 2018;50(2):77–82.

49. Davis ME, Haglund NA, Tricarico NM, et al. Development of acquired von Willebrand syndrome during short-term micro axial pump support: implications for bleeding in a patient bridged to a long-term continuous-flow left ventricular assist device. ASAIO J 2014;60(3):355–7.

50. Kalbhenn J, Schlagenhauf A, Rosenfelder S, et al. Acquired von Willebrand syndrome and impaired platelet function during venovenous extracorporeal

membrane oxygenation: rapid onset and fast recovery. J Heart Lung Transplant 2018;37(8):985–91.

51. Mohri H, Motomura S, Kanamori H, et al. Clinical significance of inhibitors in acquired von Willebrand syndrome. Blood 1998;91(10):3623–9.

52. Mohri H, Tanabe J, Yamazaki E, et al. Acquired type 2A von Willebrand disease in chronic myelocytic leukemia. Hematopathol Mol Hematol 1996;10(3):123–33.

53. Federici AB. Acquired von Willebrand syndrome: an underdiagnosed and misdiagnosed bleeding complication in patients with lymphoproliferative and myeloproliferative disorders. Semin Hematol 2006;43(1 Suppl 1):S48–58.

54. Rottenstreich A, Kleinstern G, Krichevsky S, et al. Factors related to the development of acquired von Willebrand syndrome in patients with essential thrombocythemia and polycythemia vera. Eur J Intern Med 2017;41:49–54.

55. Tefferi A, Gangat N, Wolanskyj AP. Management of extreme thrombocytosis in otherwise low-risk essential thrombocythemia; does number matter? Blood 2006;108(7):2493–4.

56. Mital A, Prejzner W, Bieniaszewska M, et al. Prevalence of acquired von Willebrand syndrome during essential thrombocythemia: a retrospective analysis of 170 consecutive patients. Pol Arch Med Wewn 2015;125(12):914–20.

57. Mital A, Prejzner W, Świątkowska-Stodulska R, et al. Factors predisposing to acquired von Willebrand syndrome during the course of polycythemia vera: retrospective analysis of 142 consecutive cases. Thromb Res 2015;136(4):754–7.

58. Federici AB, Stabile F, Castaman G, et al. Treatment of acquired von Willebrand syndrome in patients with monoclonal gammopathy of uncertain significance: comparison of three different therapeutic approaches. Blood 1998;92(8):2707–11.

59. Dicke C, Schneppenheim S, Holstein K, et al. Distinct mechanisms account for acquired von Willebrand syndrome in plasma cell dyscrasias. Ann Hematol 2016;95(6):945–57.

60. Harrison JS, Frazier SR, McConnell DD, et al. Evidence of both von Willebrand factor deposition and factor V deposition onto AL amyloid as the cause of a severe bleeding diathesis. Blood Coagul Fibrinolysis 2017;28(4):342–7.

61. Kos CA, Ward JE, Malek K, et al. Association of acquired von Willebrand syndrome with AL amyloidosis. Am J Hematol 2007;82(5):363–7.

62. Stufano F, Baronciani L, Biguzzi E, et al. Severe acquired von Willebrand syndrome secondary to systemic lupus erythematosus. Haemophilia 2019;25(1):e30–2.

63. Cao X-Y, Li M-T, Zhang X, et al. Characteristics of acquired inhibitors to factor VIII and von Willebrand factor secondary to systemic lupus erythematosus: experiences from a Chinese tertiary medical center. J Clin Rheumatol Pract Rep Rheum Musculoskelet Dis 2019. https://doi.org/10.1097/RHU.0000000000001284.

64. Taveras Alam S, Alexis K, Sridharan A, et al. Acquired von Willebrand's syndrome in systemic lupus erythematosus. Case Rep Hematol 2014;2014:208597.

65. Gavva C, Patel P, Shen Y-M, et al. A case of autoimmune severe acquired von Willebrand syndrome (type 3-like). Transfus Apher Sci 2017;56(3):431–3.

66. Dicke C, Holstein K, Schneppenheim S, et al. Acquired hemophilia A and von Willebrand syndrome in a patient with late-onset systemic lupus erythematosus. Exp Hematol Oncol 2014;3:21.

67. Viallard JF, Pellegrin JL, Vergnes C, et al. Three cases of acquired von Willebrand disease associated with systemic lupus erythematosus. Br J Haematol 1999;105(2):532–7.

68. Hong S, Lee J, Chi H, et al. Systemic lupus erythematosus complicated by acquired von Willebrand's syndrome. Lupus 2008;17(9):846–8.

69. Niiya M, Niiya K, Takazawa Y, et al. Acquired type 3-like von Willebrand syndrome preceded full-blown systemic lupus erythematosus. Blood Coagul Fibrinolysis 2002;13(4):361–5.

70. Hernández-Gilsoul T, Atisha-Fregoso Y, Vargas-Ruíz AG, et al. Pulmonary hypertension secondary to hyperviscosity in a patient with rheumatoid arthritis and acquired von Willebrand disease: a case report. J Med Case Rep 2013;7:232.

71. Martínez-Murillo C, Quintana González S, Ambriz Fernández R, et al. [Report of 2 cases with acquired von Willebrand disease and one with acquired hemophilia A]. Rev Investig Clin Organo Hosp Enfermedades Nutr 1995;47(3):211–6.

72. Lazarchick J, Green C. Acquired von Willebrand's disease following bone marrow transplantation. Ann Clin Lab Sci 1994;24(3):211–5.

73. Ingram GI, Kingston PJ, Leslie J, et al. Four cases of acquired von Willebrand's syndrome. Br J Haematol 1971;21(2):189–99.

74. Alhumood SA, Devine DV, Lawson L, et al. Idiopathic immune-mediated acquired von Willebrand's disease in a patient with angiodysplasia: demonstration of an unusual inhibitor causing a functional defect and rapid clearance of von Willebrand factor. Am J Hematol 1999;60(2):151–7.

75. Coppes MJ, Zandvoort SW, Sparling CR, et al. Acquired von Willebrand disease in Wilms' tumor patients. J Clin Oncol 1992;10(3):422–7.

76. Bruggers CS, McElligott K, Rallison ML. Acquired von Willebrand disease in twins with autoimmune hypothyroidism: response to desmopressin and L-thyroxine therapy. J Pediatr 1994;125(6 Pt 1):911–3.

77. Franchini M, de Gironcoli M, Lippi G, et al. Efficacy of desmopressin as surgical prophylaxis in patients with acquired von Willebrand disease undergoing thyroid surgery. Haemophilia 2002;8(2):142–4.

78. Michiels JJ, Schroyens W, Berneman Z, et al. Acquired von Willebrand syndrome type 1 in hypothyroidism: reversal after treatment with thyroxine. Clin Appl Thromb 2001;7(2):113–5.

79. Conrad ME, Latour LF. Acquired von Willebrand's disease, IgE polyclonal gammopathy and griseofulvin therapy. Am J Hematol 1992;41(2):143.

80. Castaman G, Lattuada A, Mannucci PM, et al. Characterization of two cases of acquired transitory von Willebrand syndrome with ciprofloxacin: evidence for heightened proteolysis of von Willebrand factor. Am J Hematol 1995;49(1):83–6.

81. Serdaroglu G, Tütüncüoglu S, Kavakli K, et al. Coagulation abnormalities and acquired von Willebrand's disease type 1 in children receiving valproic acid. J Child Neurol 2002;17(1):41–3.

82. Lazarchick J, Conroy JM. The effect of 6% hydroxyethyl starch and desmopressin infusion on von Willebrand factor: ristocetin cofactor activity. Ann Clin Lab Sci 1995;25(4):306–9.

83. Dalrymple-Hay M, Aitchison R, Collins P, et al. Hydroxyethyl starch induced acquired von Willebrand's disease. Clin Lab Haematol 1992;14(3):209–11.

84. Jonville-Béra AP, Autret-Leca E, Gruel Y. Acquired type I von Willebrand's disease associated with highly substituted hydroxyethyl starch. N Engl J Med 2001;345(8):622–3.

85. Weyand AC, James PD. Sexism in the management of bleeding disorders. Res Pract Thromb Haemost 2020;5(1):51–4.

86. Haberichter SL, Balistreri M, Christopherson P, et al. Assay of the von Willebrand factor (VWF) propeptide to identify patients with type 1 von Willebrand disease with decreased VWF survival. Blood 2006;108(10):3344–51.

87. Scott JP, Vokac EA, Schroeder T, et al. The von Willebrand factor propolypeptide, von Willebrand antigen II (vWAgII), distinguishes acquired von Willebrand syndrome (AvWS) due to decreased synthesis of von Willebrand factor (vWF) from AvWS due to increased clearance of vWF [abstract]. Blood 1995; 86(suppl):196a.

88. Randi AM, Smith KE, Castaman G. von Willebrand factor regulation of blood vessel formation. Blood 2018;132(2):132–40.

89. Starke RD, Ferraro F, Paschalaki KE, et al. Endothelial von Willebrand factor regulates angiogenesis. Blood 2011;117(3):1071–80.

90. Randi AM. Endothelial dysfunction in von Willebrand disease: angiogenesis and angiodysplasia. Thromb Res 2016;141:S55–8.

91. Castillo JJ, Gustine JN, Meid K, et al. Low levels of von Willebrand markers associate with high serum IgM levels and improve with response to therapy, in patients with Waldenström macroglobulinaemia. Br J Haematol 2019;184(6): 1011–4.

92. Franchini M, Mannucci PM. Acquired von Willebrand syndrome: focused for hematologists. Haematologica 2020;105(8):2032–7.

93. Abou-Ismail MY, Rodgers GM, Bray PF, et al. Acquired von Willebrand syndrome in monoclonal gammopathy: a scoping review on hemostatic management. Res Pract Thromb Haemost. Available at: https://onlinelibrary.wiley.com/doi/abs/10.1002/rth2.12481. Accessed February 17, 2021.

94. Mannucci PM, Lombardi R, Bader R, et al. Studies of the pathophysiology of acquired von Willebrand's disease in seven patients with lymphoproliferative disorders or benign monoclonal gammopathies. Blood 1984;64(3):614–21.

95. Franchini M, Veneri D, Lippi G. The use of recombinant activated factor VII in congenital and acquired von Willebrand disease. Blood Coagul Fibrinolysis 2006;17(8):615–9.

96. Kanakry JA, Gladstone DE. Maintaining hemostasis in acquired von Willebrand syndrome: a review of intravenous immunoglobulin and the importance of rituximab dose scheduling. Transfusion (Paris) 2013;53(8):1730–5.

97. Hawken J, Knott A, Alsakkaf W, et al. Rituximab to the rescue: novel therapy for chronic gastrointestinal bleeding due to angiodysplasia and acquired von Willebrand syndrome. Frontline Gastroenterol 2019;10(4):434–7.

98. Kurahashi H, Kawabata Y, Michishita Y, et al. [Durable remission attained with rituximab therapy in a patient with acquired von Willebrand syndrome associated with CD20-positive lymphoproliferative disorder]. Rinsho Ketsueki 2018; 59(4):420–5.

99. Pasa S, Altintas A, Cil T, et al. A case of essential mixed cryoglobulinemia and associated acquired von-Willebrand disease treated with rituximab. J Thromb Thrombolysis 2009;27(2):220–2.

100. Basnet S, Lin C, Dhital R, et al. Acquired von Willebrand disease associated with monoclonal gammopathy of unknown significance. Case Rep Oncol Med 2017; 2017:9295780.

101. Grimaldi D, Bartolucci P, Gouault-Heilmann M, et al. Rituximab failure in a patient with monoclonal gammopathy of undetermined significance (MGUS)-associated acquired von Willebrand syndrome. Thromb Haemost 2008;99(4):782–3.

102. Ojeda-Uribe M, Caron C, Itzhar-Baikian N, et al. Bortezomib effectiveness in one patient with acquired von Willebrand syndrome associated to monoclonal gammopathy of undetermined significance. Am J Hematol 2010;85(5):396.

103. Loyaga-Rendon RY, Hashim T, Tallaj JA, et al. Octreotide in the management of recurrent gastrointestinal bleed in patients supported by continuous flow left ventricular assist devices. ASAIO J 2015;61(1):107–9.

104. Shah KB, Gunda S, Emani S, et al. Multicenter evaluation of octreotide as secondary prophylaxis in patients with left ventricular assist devices and gastrointestinal bleeding. Circ Heart Fail 2017;10(11):e004500.

105. Malhotra R, Shah KB, Chawla R, et al. Tolerability and biological effects of long-acting octreotide in patients with continuous flow left ventricular assist devices. ASAIO J 2017;63(3):367–70.

106. Hayes HM, Dembo LG, Larbalestier R, et al. Management options to treat gastrointestinal bleeding in patients supported on rotary left ventricular assist devices: a single-center experience. Artif Organs 2010;34(9):703–6.

107. Draper K, Kale P, Martin B, et al. Thalidomide for treatment of gastrointestinal angiodysplasia in patients with left ventricular assist devices: case series and treatment protocol. J Heart Lung Transplant 2015;34(1):132–4.

108. Ray R, Kale PP, Ha R, et al. Treatment of left ventricular assist device-associated arteriovenous malformations with thalidomide. ASAIO J 2014;60(4):482–3.

109. Seng BJJ, Teo LLY, Chan LL, et al. Novel use of low-dose thalidomide in refractory gastrointestinal bleeding in left ventricular assist device patients. Int J Artif Organs 2017;40(11):636–40.

Secondary Hemostasis and Fibrinolysis

Hemophilia A (Factor VIII Deficiency)

Craig D. Seaman, MD, MS[a], Frederico Xavier, MD, MS[b], Margaret V. Ragni, MD, MPH[c],*

KEYWORDS

- Gene therapy • Hemarthrosis • Inhibitors • Ultrasound • Nonfactor therapy
- prophylaxis

KEY POINTS

- Genetic testing, including gene sequencing, is indicated for family planning, carrier testing, and prenatal diagnosis.
- Inhibitor assays have been adapted to measure anti-factor VIII during factor treatment and novel nonfactor therapy.
- Novel nonfactor agents and gene therapy simplify treatment, decrease bleeds, and improve clinical outcomes.

INTRODUCTION

There has been an explosion of new techniques and new therapies that are revolutionizing disease management in patients with hemophilia, significantly decreasing bleeding and improving quality of life while providing insights into the rebalancing of hemostasis. Genetic testing and next-generation sequencing have increased the number of families with an identified defect, and improved carrier testing and prenatal diagnosis. The routine use of musculoskeletal ultrasound examination in clinic has enhanced the diagnosis and management of early joint damage and hemarthroses. The pharmacokinetic measure of factor peak and trough has contributed to more effective prophylaxis and joint bleed prevention. Laboratory advances including heat treatment have improved the detection of inhibitors during factor treatment, and chromogenic assays using bovine agents have standardized inhibitor assessment during nonfactor therapy. The introduction of novel nonfactor therapies has simplified

[a] Department of Medicine, Division Hematology/Oncology, University of Pittsburgh Medical Center, 3636 Boulevard of the Allies, Pittsburgh, PA 15213-4306, USA; [b] Department of Pediatrics, Division Hematology/Oncology, University of Pittsburgh Medical Center, Children's Hospital of Pittsburgh, 4401 Penn Avenue, Pittsburgh, PA 15224, USA; [c] Medicine and Clinical Translational Research, Department of Medicine, Division Hematology/Oncology, University of Pittsburgh Medical Center, Hemophilia Center of Western Pennsylvania, 3636 Boulevard of the Allies, Pittsburgh, PA 15213-4306, USA
* Corresponding author.
E-mail address: ragni@pitt.edu

Hematol Oncol Clin N Am 35 (2021) 1117–1129
https://doi.org/10.1016/j.hoc.2021.07.006
0889-8588/21/© 2021 Elsevier Inc. All rights reserved.
hemonc.theclinics.com

treatment, decreased bleeding rates, and improved quality of life. Gene therapy trials have provided the potential for a 1-shot phenotypic "cure," providing hope for those in resource-poor countries where factor is scarce.

CLINICAL ASPECTS OF DISEASE
Genetic Assessment

Hemophilia A is an X-linked recessive disorder caused by a deficiency in factor VIII (FVIII). The FVIII gene is located on the long arm of the X chromosome (Xq28). It is 187 kilobases (kb) in size and composed of 26 exons. The resulting messenger RNA is approximately 9 kb and encodes a mature protein of 2332 amino acids.[1] Almost two-thirds of hemophilia A cases are due to single nucleotide variants, most often missense mutations. Other common disease-causing pathogenic variants include deletions, which are responsible for almost one-quarter of cases, and duplications.[2] The type of mutation predicts the severity of disease. Those that result in significant disruption of the FVIII protein, such as deletions and nonsense mutations, are associated with severe disease, whereas mild and moderate disease are more commonly seen with missense mutations.[3] The intron 22 inversion is the most common mutation, accounting for 20% of all types of hemophilia A and 45% of mutations in severe hemophilia A.[4]

Hemophilia A affects 1 in 5000 live male births.[5] Among female carriers, there is a 50% chance of having an affected son or carrier daughter. All female offspring of affected males are obligate carriers, whereas no male offspring are affected. Depending on the degree of X chromosome lyonization, some female carriers are symptomatic. Although a family history is often present, spontaneous mutations occurs in one-third of hemophilia cases.[6]

Genetic assessment should be offered to all affected patients (probands), obligate carriers, and at-risk female relatives, because it may provide valuable disease information regarding inhibitor risk,[7] immune tolerance response,[8] and targeted FVIII gene sequencing in at-risk female relatives. Ideally, the causative genetic variant should be identified first in the proband or obligate carrier, after which other at-risk carriers can be evaluated. Because carriers may be asymptomatic or have normal FVIII levels, genetic assessment is essential to determine carrier status.[9] In probands, genetic testing should be directed by disease severity.[10] In severe hemophilia A, the intron 22 inversion mutation is assessed first, but if negative, followed sequentially by intron 1 inversion assessment, FVIII coding region analysis, and copy number variants. FVIII gene analysis is recommended in moderate and mild disease and in at-risk carriers where the familial genetic variant is unknown. Otherwise, FVIII gene sequencing is performed by polymerase chain reaction and Sanger sequencing or next-generation sequencing.[11]

Genetic counseling should be provided by a genetic counselor regarding tests performed, the rationale, limitations, potential consequences, and an explanation of testing results.[12] In pregnant carriers, prenatal counseling should include discussion of prenatal diagnosis of male fetuses, preimplantation genetic diagnosis, management of pregnancy and delivery,[13,14] and chorionic villus sampling, amniocentesis, delivery, preimplantation diagnosis, and termination.

Laboratory Diagnosis and Monitoring

The diagnosis of hemophilia A is suspected by clinical history of bleeding and/or family history. In a suspected patient, initial laboratory testing should include platelet count, activated partial thromboplastin time (aPTT), and prothrombin time. Patients with hemophilia A will have a prolonged aPTT, normal prothrombin time, and normal platelet count (**Table 1**). If the aPTT is prolonged, a mixing study in which patient plasma is mixed 1:1 with pooled normal plasma is done to determine if factor deficiency or inhibitor is present.[15] If the aPTT corrects, a factor deficiency is suspected. If factor deficiency is suspected, factor activity levels are performed by 1-stage clotting assays.[16] Another method to measure FVIII activity is the chromogenic assay, in which FVIII is the rate-limiting step in FXa production and the amount of FXa produced is proportional to FVIII activity as determined by color intensity.[17] The 1-stage and chromogenic FVIII assays may be slightly discrepant, for example, overestimating FVIII levels in moderate or mild hemophilia[18] or with use of extended half-life products.[19]

FVIII inhibitor assays are determined by the Bethesda assay in which normal pooled plasma is mixed 1:1 with diluted plasma, an imidazole buffer, and normal pooled plasma as the source of FVIII.[20] The inhibitor is measured in Bethesda units with 1 Bethesda unit defined as the amount of inhibitor that neutralizes 50% of residual FVIII activity after a 2-hour incubation at 37 °C. The Nijmegen modification of this assay, in which FVIII-deficient plasma replaces the imidazole buffer, improves the sensitivity and specificity of the Bethesda assay and provides for the detection of low-titer inhibitors.[21] A chromogenic assay may also improve detection of low-titer inhibitors in those using nonfactor agents that interfere with the assay.[22] A heat neutralization modification of the Bethesda assay, in which the plasma sample is warmed to 56 °C for 30 minutes, enables the measure of inhibitors in those concurrently receiving factor concentrate.[23]

Finally, some novel nonfactor agents, that is, emicizumab, may affect aPTT-based assays, including the 1-stage FVIII assay, because, in contrast with FVIII, emicizumab does not require activation by thrombin, the major rate-limiting step. Thus, at very low concentrations of this drug, the aPTT may be normal[24] and the 1-stage FVIII assay may be elevated.[25] Emicizumab also interferes in the chromogenic assays of FVIII and FVIII antibody assay.[26–28] For that reason, a chromogenic FVIII and anti-FVIII assays using bovine components, to which the drug is insensitive, are recommended.

Acute Bleeds

Hemophilia severity is stratified by the risk of bleeding according to factor activity levels, with 3 risk levels: mild, moderate, and severe.[29] The accuracy of such a classification is limited, because patients with severe deficiencies, for example, may have mild bleeding phenotypes. The goal of acute bleed management is to achieve a recommended hemostatic level to stop bleeding and to provide hemostasis during recovery to avoid rebleeding. The hemostatic level desired is based on the severity and site of bleeding, as recommended by guidance from the World Federation of Hemophilia[10] and National Hemophilia Foundation.[30]

Most bleeds occur in joints and muscles. Confirmation of a joint or muscle bleed is by point-of-care ultrasound examination or more sophisticated imaging.

Table 1 Coagulation tests in hemophilia A		
Screening Tests	**FVIII Assays**	**FVIII Inhibitor Assays**
Platelet count	One-stage assay	Bethesda assay
Partial thromboplastin time	Chromogenic assay	Nijmegen Bethesda assay
	Bovine chromogenic assay	Chromogenic Bethesda assay
Prothrombin time		Bovine chromogenic Bethesda assay

Importantly, factor replacement therapy is given before imaging or laboratory assessment, because a delay may result in uncontrolled bleeding and poor outcomes. In general, a 10% to 20% level is recommended for mild bleeds, 20% to 50% for moderate bleeds, 50% to 80% for severe bleeds, and more than 100% for life-threatening bleeds. For patients with mild disease, desmopressin is the preferred hemostatic agent. Adjunctive therapy includes protection, rest, ice/cold compresses, compression, and elevation; pain management; and antifibrinolytic agents (eg, tranexamic acid and/or epsilon aminocaproic acid). Early rehabilitation is recommended after bleed resolution. A multidisciplinary approach with a physical therapist, rehabilitation specialist, and pain management expert is recommended. The duration of the treatment varies with the bleed severity and location and is tailored to avoid the risk of rebleeding, especially when resuming normal activity after a bleed or with physical therapy. A pain management plan is also critical to management. Response is assessed as excellent, good, moderate, or none (**Table 2**). Intracranial hemorrhage and central nervous system bleeding should be suspected in those sustaining head trauma, whiplash injuries, new hypertension, prolonged headaches, a change in mental status, or severe back pain, or in children with lethargy, fussiness, or inconsolable crying.[31–33] Spontaneous bleeds may occur at any age.[34] The initial management should aim for clotting factor replacement up to 100% correction for the next 7 days, followed by 50% correction for 10 to 14 days.[33,34]

Muscle bleeds are aggressively managed to avoid rebleeding. To limit injury or worsening of bleeds during physical therapy, active rather than passive range of motion is advised. Aggressive factor replacement is indicated for bleeds in a muscle compartment. If the risk of rebleeding is higher, particularly in very active patients, a prolonged course with a more aggressive replacement dosing (50%–80%) is preferred, with follow-up by a physical therapist familiar with point-of-care ultrasound examination. In general, 3 consecutive days of factor replacement to achieve 60% to 80% activity is recommended, followed by 50% levels daily or every other day until the pain subsides. Factor is usually continued until resolution of the bleed, preferably confirmed by point-of-care ultrasound examination, after which physiotherapy with isometric exercises may begin.[35]

Mucocutaneous bleeds generally require, in addition to factor, cauterization for recurrent epistaxis or adjuvant antifibrinolytic or local hemostatic therapy, for example, Gelfoam, for dental or surgical evaluation. Intestinal bleeding requires more aggressive factor management to maintain the blood volume and a stable hemoglobin. The duration of therapy is based on time to local healing, for example, cessation of hematochezia or melena.

Table 2	
Response of acute hemarthrosis to standard half-life factor replacement	
Excellent	Complete pain relief and resolution of bleeding within 8 h of infusion, with no further factor infusion after 72 h
Good	Significant pain relief or improvement in bleeding within 8 h of infusion but requiring >1 dose of factor replacement within 72 h for complete resolution.
Moderate	Modest pain relief or improvement in signs of bleeding within 8 h of infusion and requiring >1 infusion within 72 h without complete resolution.
None	No or minimal improvement or worsening within 8 h of the initial infusion.

Hemarthrosis

More than 80% of patients with severe hemophilia A experience spontaneous hematomas and hemarthroses. Despite advances in management, hemarthrosis is still a major cause of morbidity and health care cost, and often the first bleeding manifestation primarily in large joints, the elbow, knee, and ankle. When bleeds recur in the same target joint, irreversible hemophilic arthropathy may occur. If disability and pain progress, joint replacement may be required.

The extravasation of blood into the synovial space during hemarthrosis leads to an inflammatory response owing to the presence of iron and generation of iron-catalyzed reactive oxygen intermediates. Although transient in initial bleeds,[36] the inflammatory response may become chronic with repetitive bleeds and lead to permanent damage and degeneration of the joint cartilage, in association with cytokine elaboration promoted by macrophages, B lymphocytes, T lymphocytes, and mast cells. Among these, IL-1beta and tumor necrosis factor-alpha, enhanced IL-6, and protected by IL-10, IL-4, and anti–IL-6.[37,38] There is increasing interest in targeting cytokines to decrease hemophilic arthropathy, for example, IL-1 inhibitors.[39]

Prophylaxis

In addition to early factor replacement to treat acute bleeds, robust evidence supports joint bleed prevention or prophylaxis, that is, the regular infusion of clotting protein to prevent joint bleeds. Prophylaxis prevents, halts, or decelerates the development of hemophilic arthropathy (primary, secondary, or tertiary prophylaxis).[40] Prophylaxis is initiated in severe hemophilia by age 2, and typically after the first episode of hemarthrosis.[29] Because the clinical response is variable, individualized prophylaxis regimens based on peak and trough FVIII levels are recommended. Although a trough level of 3% was the previous goal of prophylaxis, recent evidence suggests higher that trough levels are necessary to decrease bleeds and joint damage.[41,42] The web-accessible app based on population pharmacokinetics (WAPPS-hemo) has been widely adopted to tailor individualized prophylaxis dosing.[43] Recently, the use of nonfactor therapy, for example, emicuzimab, has dramatically decreased bleeds and simplified treatment, but questions remain regarding its optimal use in prophylaxis[44] and inhibitor management.[45]

Inhibitors

Inhibitor formation to FVIII is among the most serious challenges of hemophilia treatment. Inhibitors are T-cell–dependent B-cell responses to exogenous FVIII[46] that occur in 30% of those with severe hemophilia A, rendering factor treatment ineffective and leading to poorly controlled bleeds, with high morbidity,[47] hospitalization,[48] and costs.[49] Although the risk factors for inhibitor formation are established, that is, large deletion mutations, race, and family history,[50] the major risk is FVIII exposure and the intensity of FVIII exposure.[51] It is hypothesized that frequent, intense FVIII exposure leads to immune activation and the danger response, with immune system activation and an immune response directed at the large FVIII molecule.[52]

Once an inhibitor is detected, management requires a 2-fold approach: (1) acute bleed management, with recombinant FVIIa or activated prothrombin complex concentrate and (2) immune tolerance induction with daily high-dose FVIII.[53,54] Although 80% of patients achieve tolerance, the burden is high, requiring 12 months or more of daily factor and, in most, port placement with its associated infection risk. Thus, a major goal of hemophilia management is to prevent and eradicate inhibitors.[55,56] With the licensure of emicizumab, a nonfactor therapy that avoids FVIII exposure by subcutaneous administration, it is anticipated that inhibitor formation may be better managed; this modality is currently under study in several clinical trials (**Table 3**).

Table 3
Clinical trials to prevent and eradicate hemophilia inhibitors

Title	Type Study	NCT	Sample Size	Target Group	Age	Study Arms	Primary End Point

Nuwiq ITI Trial
Sponsor: Genentech
	Prospective
	Nonrandomized Trial
		04030052	N = 60	HA PUPs
				HA-I
				PTPs
					<3 y
					<21 y
						Emicizumab +
						  low-dose rFVIII
						Emicizumab +
						  low-dose rFVIII ITI
							Inhibitor Formation at 36 wk
							Inhibitor Eradication at 36 wk

INHIBIT Platform Trial 1. Inhibitor Prevention Trial 2. Inhibitor Eradication Trial Sponsor: HRSA	Prospective RCT Prospective RCT	04303559 04303572	N = 66 N = 90	HA PUPs HA-I PTPs	≥4 mo All ages	Eloctate weekly vs Emicizumab weekly Eloctate ITI qod + Emicizumab weekly vs Eloctate ITI qod	Inhibitor Formation at 48 wk Inhibitor Eradication at 48 wk
MOTIVATE Trial Sponsor: Octapharma	Observational prospective study	04023019	N = 120	HA-I PTPs	All ages	ITI alone vs Emicizumab + ITI vs Emicizumab + no ITI	Inhibitor eradication at ≤5 y

PRIORITY Trial
Sponsor: Grifols
	Prospective RCT	04621916	N = 52	Tolerized HA-I	≤12 y	Emicizumab +
						  FVIII Weekly
						  Vs
						  Emicizumab
							Inhibitor Recurrence at 96 wk

Abbreviations: HA, hemophilia A; HA-I, hemophilia A with inhibitor; ITI, immune tolerance induction; NCT, ClinicalTrials; gov identifier; pdFVIII, plasma-derived factor VIII; PUPs, previously untreated patients; PTPs, previously treated patients; qod, every other day; RCT, randomized controlled trial; rFVIII, recombinant factor VIII.

Table 4
Novel therapies in hemophilia

Novel Agent	Mechanism	Target Population	Route	Dosing	Complications
BIVV001	VIII-VWF-Fc-fusion protein	Hemophilia A	IV	Weekly	Poor compliance Port-related infection
Emicizumab	Bispecific monoclonal antibody, FVIII mimic	Hemophilia A with or without Inhibitors	SQ	Weekly or biweekly or monthly	Injection site reactions Thrombosis
Fitusiran	Small interfering RNA antithrombin knockdown	Hemophilia A with or without inhibitors	SQ	Monthly or bimonthly	Injection site reactions Thrombosis
Concizumab	Anti-tissue factor pathway inhibitor monoclonal antibody	Hemophilia A with or without inhibitors	SQ	Daily	Injection site reactions
Adenoviral-associated viral FVIII	Adenoviral-associated viral B-domain–deleted FVIII vector-gene therapy	Hemophilia A	IV	Single dose	Immune responses Level variability Waning levels Hepatotoxicity

NOVEL APPROACHES TO HEMOSTATIC MANAGEMENT

There has been an explosion of novel therapeutics for hemophilia A with or without inhibitors that decrease bleeds more effectively than factor therapies (**Table 4**). These agents provide simpler, more durable administration. The first of these is the novel BIVV001, in which FVIII is bound to VWF through an XTEN linker, providing steric protection for FVIII in the circulation. This modification improves the half-life of FVIII to allow weekly dosing by the intravenous route,[57] a major improvement over the current 2 to 3 times per week with FVIII therapies. The drug is well-tolerated and clinical trials continue in adults and children.

Novel Nonfactor Therapies

Nonfactor therapies include the bispecific monoclonal antibody FVIII mimetic, emicizumab,[58,59] the small interfering RNA antithrombin knockdown, fitusiran,[60] and the anti–tissue factor pathway inhibitor concizumab,[61] each administered subcutaneously, achieving better hemostasis than with standard factor. Emicizumab is the only agent licensed by the US Food and Drug Administration and has been shown in postlicensure studies to be as effective in patients with and without inhibitors,[62] with low rates of breakthrough bleeds and with improved health ratings in 85% of patients. It is also effective in surgery, when factor is given preoperatively and for the first few postoperatively, and tapered over several weeks.[63] The use of activated prothrombin complex concentrates in combination with emicizumab should be avoided, because these agents may result in thrombotic micriangiopathy.[62] In fact, the unexpected occurrence of thrombosis during clinical trials of all 3 therapies underscores the fine line between hemostasis and thrombosis; the potential risk in hemophilia patients who are obese, hypertensive, or diabetic; and need for biomarkers to predict thrombosis.

Gene Therapy

Hemophilia A gene therapy involves a single intravenous administration of a human B-domain–deleted FVIII gene encapsulated in an adenoviral-associated viral (AAV) vector. This AAV–human FVIII targets the hepatocyte, with subsequent FVIII synthesis and secretion into the circulation to achieve 1-time phenotypic cure. In several trials, AAV–human FVIII has led to a 90% decrease in spontaneous bleeds and factor use.[64,65] Although FVIII activity levels have ranged from 10% to 50% or higher, there remain concerns, including immune response to the vector, hepatotoxicity, and variable and waning FVIII levels. The latter is attributed to targeting the hepatocyte, rather than liver sinusoidal endothelial cells where FVIII is synthesized, leading to endoplasmic reticulum stress owing to the large size of FVIII.[66] Despite these issues, FVIII gene therapy has the potential to improve health outcomes in resource-poor settings where factor is scarce, and several analyses have shown gene therapy is cost effective when balanced against lifetime costs of factor, hospitalization, morbidity, and disability.[67,68]

SUMMARY

The field of hemophilia is rapidly changing. Pharmacokinetic studies provide for personalized prophylaxis to optimize bleed reduction and joint damage. Novel nonfactor therapeutics have simplified prophylaxis and bleed prevention in those with and without inhibitors. Clinical trials are evaluating these agents in the prevention and eradication of inhibitors. The recognition of thrombosis with nonfactor therapies, although unexpected, points to need for biomarkers of risk to assure patient safety.

Gene therapy with AAV vector gene administration promises a single-dose phenotypic cure, and although it may hold promise in resource-poor settings, much needs to be learned about the mechanism of waning factor levels and hepatotoxicity. Despite these setbacks, technological advances are expected to enhance our understanding of coagulation improve clinical outcomes and quality of life in those with hemophilia.

CLINICS CARE POINTS

Treatment Plan
- Ensure that affected patients have a written treatment plan, including dose, dose frequency, and product.
- Ensure the treatment plan is available in an emergency room setting, for bleeds, trauma, or surgery.
- Ensure factor is available for acute or traumatic bleed treatment.

Genetic Testing
- Incorporate genetic testing and family history into the care plan for every patient with hemophilia.
- Use genetic testing to screen female relatives of affected patients, not known to be obligate carriers.

Prophylaxis

- Initiate prophylaxis early, preferably after 1 to 2 spontaneous joint bleeds to limit joint disease.
- Perform pharmacokinetic peak and trough factor levels to ensure optimal prophylaxis.

Hemarthrosis
- Use musculoskeletal ultrasound examination to establish early joint disease and follow treatment.

Nonfactor Therapy
- Use nonfactor therapy as prophylaxis to prevent bleeds; use factor to treat acute bleeds.

Laboratory Assays
- Obtain cord blood on male offspring at delivery for factor levels to determine diagnosis.
- Use the heat-treated Nijmegen anti-VIII assay to avoid impact of factor treatment for inhibitor testing.
- Use chromogenic bovine reagent assays to measure factor and inhibitor during emicizumab therapy.

Thrombosis
- Assess thrombotic risk factors, for example, obesity and hypertension, before initiating nonfactor therapy.
- For acute bleed management during nonfactor therapy, limit factor to the minimum necessary treatment.
- Avoid activated prothrombin complex concentrates in those receiving emicizumab.
- Educate patients regarding symptoms and signs of thrombosis.

DISCLOSURE STATEMENT

Dr Ragni reports institutional research funding and advisory board fees from Alnylam, BioMarin, Bioverativ, Spark Therapeutics, and Takeda Pharmaceuticals, and institutional research funding from Sangamo. Dr Seaman reports institutional research funding from Bioverativ and consulting fees from Bayer Pharmaceuticals, Genentech, HEMA Biologics, Sanofi Genzyme, Spark Therapeutics, and Takeda Pharmaceuticals. Dr Xavier reports institutional research funding from Bioverativ and advisory board fees from Genentech.

REFERENCES

1. Al-Allaf FA, Taher MM, Abduljaleel Z, et al. Molecular analysis of factor VIII and factor IX gene in hemophilia patients: identification of novel mutations and molecular dynamics studies. J Clin Med Res 2017;9:317–31.
2. Swystun LL, James PD. Genetic diagnosis in hemophilia and von Willebrand disease. Blood Rev 2017;31:47–56.
3. Pruthi R. Hemophilia: a practical approach to genetic testing. Mayo Clin Proc 2005;80:1485–99.
4. Dutta D, Gunasekera D, Ragni MV, et al. Accurate, simple, and inexpensive assays to diagnosis F8 gene inversion mutations in hemophilia A patients and carriers. Blood Adv 2016;1:231–9.
5. Soucie JM, Jackson EB, Jackson D. Occurrence of hemophilia in the United States. The Hemophilia Surveillance System Project Investigators. Am J Hematol 1998;59:288–94.
6. Kulkarni R, Soucie JM, Lusher J, et al. Sites of initial bleeding episodes, mode of delivery and age of diagnosis in babies with haemophilia diagnosed before the age of 2 years: a report from the Centers for Disease Control and Prevention's (CDC) Universal Data Collection (UDC) project. Haemophilia 2009;15:1281–90.
7. Gouw SC, van den Berg HM, Oldenburg J, et al. F8 gene mutation type and inhibitor development in patients with severe hemophilia A: systematic review and meta-analysis. Blood 2012;119:2922–34.
8. Coppola A, Margaglione M, Santagostino E, et al. Factor VIII gene (F8) mutations as predictors of outcome in immune tolerance induction of hemophilia A patients with high- responding inhibitors. J Thromb Haemost 2009;7:1809–15.
9. James PD, Mahlangu J, Bidlingmaier C, et al. Evaluation of the utility of the ISTH-BAT in haemophilia carriers: a multinational study. Haemophilia 2016;22:912–8.
10. Srivastava A, Santagostino E, Dougall A, et al. WFH guidelines for the management of hemophilia, 3rd edition. Haemophilia 2020;26(Suppl 6):1–158.
11. Johnsen JM, Fletcher SN, Huston H, et al. Novel approach to genetic analysis and results in 3000 hemophilia patients enrolled in the My Life, Our Future initiative. Blood Adv 2017;1:824–34.
12. Gomez K, Laffan M, Keeney S, et al. Recommendations for the clinical interpretation of genetic variants and presentation of results to patients with inherited bleeding disorders: a UK Haemophilia Centre Doctors' Organisation Good Practice Paper. Haemophilia 2019;25:116–26.
13. Zarrilli F, Sanna V, Ingino R, et al. Prenatal diagnosis of haemophilia: our experience of 44 cases. Clin Chem Lab Med 2013;51:2233–8.
14. Chen M, Chang SP, Ma GC, et al. Preimplantation genetic diagnosis of hemophilia A. Thromb J 2016;14(Suppl 1):33.
15. Favaloro EJ. Coagulation mixing studies: Utility, algorithmic strategies and limitations for lupus anticoagulant testing or follow up of abnormal coagulation tests. Am J Hematol 2020;1:117–28.
16. Kitchen S, Signer-Romero K, Key NS. Current laboratory practices in the diagnosis and management of haemophilia: a global assessment. Haemophilia 2015;21:550–7.
17. Baker P, Platton S, Gibson C, et al. Guidelines on the laboratory aspects of assays used in haemostasis and thrombosis. Br J Hematol 2020;191:347–62.
18. Potgieter JJ, Damgaard M, Hillarp A. One-stage vs. chromogenic assays in haemophilia A. Eur J Haematol 2015;94:38–44.

19. Young GA, Perry DJ, International Prophylaxis Study Group (IPSG). Laboratory assay measurement of modified clotting factor concentrates: a review of the literature and recommendations for practice. J Thromb Haemost 2019;17:567–73.

20. Miller CH. Laboratory testing for factor VIII and IX inhibitors in haemophilia: a review. Haemophilia 2018;24:186–97.

21. Duncan E, Collecutt M, Street A. Nijmegen-Bethesda assay to measure factor VIII inhibitors. Methods Mol Biol 2013;992:321–30.

22. Miller CH, Rice AS, Boylan B, et al. Comparison of clot-based, chromogenic, and fluorescence assays for measurement of factor VIII inhibitors in the U.S. Hemophilia Inhibitor Research Study. J Thromb Haemost 2013;11:1300–9.

23. Miller CH, Platt SJ, Kelly F, et al. Validation of Nijmegen-Bethesda assay modifications to allow inhibitor measurement during replacement therapy and facilitate inhibitor surveillance. J Thromb Haemost 2012;10:1055–61.

24. Shima M, Hanabusa H, Taki M, et al. Factor VIII-mimetic function of humanized bispecific antibody in hemophilia A. N Engl J Med 2016;374:2044–53.

25. Al-Samkari H, Croteau SE. Shifting landscape of hemophilia therapy: implications for current clinical laboratory coagulation assays. Am J Hematol 2018;93: 1082–90.

26. Adamkewicz JI, Chen DC, Paz-Priel I. Effects and interferences of emicizumab, a humanised bispecific antibody mimicking activated factor VIII cofactor function, on coagulation assays. Thromb Haemost 2019;119:1084–93.

27. Tripodi A, Chantarangkul V, Novembrino C, et al. Emicizumab, the factor VIII mimetic bispecific monoclonal antibody and its measure in plasma. Clin Chem Lab Med 2020;59:365–71.

28. Muller J, Pekrul I, Potzsch B, et al. Laboratory monitoring in emicizumab-treated persons with hemophilia A. Thromb Haemost 2019;119:1384–93.

29. Blanchette VS, Key NS, Ljung LR, et al. for the Subcommittee on Factor VIII, Factor IX and Rare Coagulation Disorders. Definitions in hemophilia: communication from the SSC of the ISTH. J Thromb Haemost 2014;12:1935–9.

30. Medical and Scientific Advisory Committee (MASAC). Guidelines for emergency department management of individuals with hemophilia and other bleeding disorders. Natl Hemophilia Found 2014;257.

31. Ljung RC. Intracranial haemorrhage in haemophilia A and B. Br J Haematol 2008; 140:378–84.

32. Nagel K, Pai M, Paes K, et al. Diagnosis and treatment of intracranial hemorrhage in children with hemophilia. Blood Coagul Fibrinolysis 2013;24:23–7.

33. Nakar C, Cooper DL, DiMichele D. Recombinant activated factor VII safety and efficacy in the treatment of cranial haemorrhage in patients with congenital haemophilia with inhibitors: an analysis of the Hemophilia Thrombosis Research Society Registry (2004-2008). Haemophilia 2010;16:625–31.

34. Kulkarni R, Lusher JM. Intracranial and extracranial hemorrhages in newborns with hemophilia: a review of the literature. J Pediatr Hematol Oncol 1999;289–95.

35. Strike K, Mulder K, Michael R. Exercise in haemophilia. Cochrane Database Syst Rev Rev 2016;12:1–55.

36. Hooiveld M, Roosendaal G, Vianen M, et al. Blood-induced joint damage: long-term effects in vitro and in vivo. J Rheumatol 2003;30:339–44.

37. van Meegeren ME, Roosendaal G, Jansen NWD, et al. IL-4 alone and in combination with IL-10 protects against blood-induced cartilage damage. Osteoarthr Cartil 2012;20:764–72.

38. Narkbunnam N, Sun J, Hu G, et al. IL-6 receptor antagonist as adjunctive therapy with clotting factor replacement to protect against bleeding-induced arthropathy in hemophilia. J Thromb Haemost 2013;11:881–93.

39. van Vulpen LF, Schutgens REG, Coeleveld K, et al. IL-1beta, in contrast to TNFalpha, is pivotal in blood-induced cartilage damage and is a potential target for therapy. Blood 2015;126:2239–46.

40. Manco-Johnson MJ, Abshire TC, Shapiro AD, et al. Prophylaxis versus episodic treatment to prevent joint disease in boys with severe hemophilia. N Engl J Med 2007;357:535–44.

41. Petrini P, Valentino LA, Gringeri A, et al. Individualizing prophylaxis in hemophilia: a review. Exp Rev Hematol 2015;8:237–46.

42. Ragni MV, Croteau S, Morfini M, et al. Pharmacokinetics and the transition to extended half-life factor concentrates: communication from the SSC of the ISTH. J Thromb Haemost 2018;16:1437–41.

43. McEneny-King A, Yeung CHT, Edginton AN, et al. Clinical application of Web Accessible Population Pharmacokinetic Service—Hemophilia (WAPPS-Hemo): patterns of blood sampling and patient characteristics among clinician users. Haemophilia 2020;26:56–63.

44. Malec LM, Cheng D, Witmer CM, et al. The impact of extended half-life factor concentrates on prophylaxis for severe hemophilia in the United States. Am J Hematol 2020;95:960–5.

45. Ebbert PT, Xavier F, Malec LM, et al. Observational study of recombinant factor VIII-Fc, rFVIIIFc, in hemophilia A. Thromb Res 2020;195:51–4.

46. Ragni MV, Bontempo FA, Lewis JH. Disappearance of inhibitor to factor VIII in HIV- infected hemophiliacs with progression to AIDS or severe ARC. Transfusion 1989;29:447–9.

47. Walsh CE, Soucie JM, Miller CH. Impact of inhibitors on hemophilia A mortality in the United States. Am J Hematol 2015;90:400–5.

48. Soucie JM, Symons J, Evatt B, et al. Home-based infusion therapy and hospitalization for bleeding complications among males with hemophilia. Haemophilia 2001;7:198–206.

49. Goudemand J. Pharmacoeconomic aspects of inhibitor treatment. Eur J Haematol 1998;63:24–7.

50. Ragni MV, Ojeifo O, Hill K, et al. The Hemophilia Inhibitor Study Group: risk factors for inhibitor formation in hemophilia; A prevalent case-control study. Haemophilia 2009;15:1074–82.

51. Gouw S, van den Berg HM, Fischer K, et al. Intensity of factor VIII treatment and inhibitor development in children with severe hemophilia A: the RODIN study. Blood 2013;121:4046–55.

52. Matzinger P. The danger model: a renewed sense of self. Science 2002;296: 301–5.

53. Ragni MV, Berntorp E, Carcao M, et al. Inhibitors to clotting factor. In: Srivastava A, Santagastino E, Dougall A, et al. WFH Guidelines for the management of hemophilia. Haemophilia 2020;26(Suppl 6):95–107.

54. Hay CRM, DiMichele DM. International Immune Tolerance Study: the principal results of the International Immune Tolerance Study: a randomized dose comparison. Blood 2012;119:1335–44.

55. Ragni MV, George LA. The national blueprint for future factor VIII inhibitor clinical trials: NHLBI State of the Science (SOS) Workshop on factor VIII inhibitors. Haemophilia 2019;25:581–9.

56. Bertolet M, Brooks M, Ragni MV. The design for Bayesian platform trials to prevent and eradicate inhibitors in patients with hemophilia. Blood Adv 2020;4:5433–44.
57. Konkle BA, Shapiro AD, Quon DV, et al. BIVV001: BIVV001 fusion protein as factor VIII replacement therapy for hemophilia A. N Engl J Med 2020;383:1018–27.
58. Oldenburg J, Mahlangu JN, Kim B, et al. Emicizumab prophylaxis in hemophilia A with inhibitors. N Engl J Med 2017;377:809–18.
59. Mahlangu J, Oldenburg J, Paz-Priel I, et al. Emicizumab prophylaxis in patients who have hemophilia A without inhibitors. N Engl J Med 2018;379:811–22.
60. Pasi KJ, Rangarajan S, Georgiev P, et al. Targeting of anti-thrombin in hemophilia A or B with RNAi therapy. N Engl J Med 2017;377:819–28.
61. Shapiro A, Angshaisuksiri P, Astermark J, et al. Subcutaneous concizumab prophylaxis in hemophilia A and hemophilia A/B with inhibitors: phase 2 trial results. Blood 2019;134:1973–82.
62. Ebbert PT, Xavier F, Seaman CD, et al. Emicizumab prophylaxis in hemophilia A with and without inhibitors. Haemophilia 2020;26:41–6.
63. Seaman CD, Ragni MV. Emicizumab use in major orthopedic surgery. Blood Adv 2019;3:1722–4.
64. Rangarajan S, Walsh L, Lester W, et al. AAV5-factor VIII gene transfer in severe hemophilia A. N Engl J Med 2017;377:2519–30.
65. Pasi KJ, Rangarajan S, Mitchell N, et al. Multiyear follow-up of AAV5-hFVIII-SQ gene therapy for hemophilia A. N Engl J Med 2020;382:29–40.
66. Poothong J, Pottekat A, Siirin M, et al. Factor VIII exhibits chaperone-dependent and glucose-regulated reversible amyloid formation in the endoplasmic reticulum. Blood 2020;135:1899–911.
67. Machin N, Ragni MV, Smith KJ. Gene therapy in hemophilia A: a cost-effectiveness analysis. Blood Adv 2018;2:1792–8.
68. Rind DM, Walton SM, Agboola F, et al. Valoctocogene and emicizumab for hemophilia effectiveness and value: evidence report. Institute for clinical and economic review. https://icer-review.org/material/hemophilia-a-update-evidence-report/. [Accessed 16 October 2020].

Acquired Hemophilia A

Menaka Pai, MSc, MD, FRCPC[1]

KEYWORDS

- Hemophilia • Inhibitor • Bleeding disorder • aPTT • Acquired hemophilia A

KEY POINTS

- Acquired hemophilia A is a potentially severe bleeding disorder caused by antibodies against the patient's own factor VIII.
- Bleeding in acquired hemophilia A can be spontaneous and severe.
- The clinical and laboratory presentation of acquired hemophilia A can be confused with other coagulopathies.
- The 1:1 mix can be a useful way of differentiating factor deficiency from inhibitors when faced with an isolated elevation of the activated partial thromboplastin time. However in acquired hemophilia A, inhibitor activity is time and temperature dependent, so the effect on the 1:1 mix is most evident when samples are intubated.
- Treatment involves control of bleeding and eradication of the inhibitor. Clinicians should be alert for side effects of eradicating therapies.

INTRODUCTION

Acquired hemophilia A is a bleeding disorder caused by antibodies to factor VIII (FVIII). These antibodies—called *inhibitors*—interfere with normal hemostasis, leading to potentially catastrophic bleeding. Acquired hemophilia A is a rare disease, and there is a paucity of randomized trial data to guide its treatment. However, understanding the pathogenesis and presentation of acquired hemophilia A can help clinicians to detect this severe bleeding disorder early and manage it in an evidence-based fashion.

NATURE OF THE PROBLEM

Acquired inhibitors have been reported for all coagulation factors, but by far the most common acquired inhibitor is the FVIII antibody—the inhibitor that causes acquired hemophilia A.[1,2]

McMaster University, Hamilton, Canada; Hamilton Health Sciences, Hamilton, Canada; Hamilton Regional Laboratory Medicine Program, Hamilton, Canada
[1] Room 1-270A, Hamilton General Hospital, 237 Barton Street East, Hamilton, Ontario, Canada L8L 2X2.
E-mail address: mpai@mcmaster.ca

Hematol Oncol Clin N Am 35 (2021) 1131–1142
https://doi.org/10.1016/j.hoc.2021.07.007
0889-8588/21/© 2021 Elsevier Inc. All rights reserved.

hemonc.theclinics.com

FVIII is synthesized as a 330-kDa precursor protein composed of a heavy chain and a light chain[3] (**Fig. 1**). After proteolytic cleavage, FVIII binds to the phospholipid components of platelets and endothelial cells, and to other clotting factors. The antibodies that cause acquired hemophilia A tend to be IgG antibodies that interfere with FVIII binding to factor X and factor IXa, or that interfere with FVIII binding to phospholipid and von Willebrand factor.[3–6]

Acquired FVIII inhibitors show type II or second-order kinetics, inactivating FVIII in a nonlinear fashion[7–9] (**Fig. 2**). Initially, inactivation is rapid, but it then slows to an equilibrium. The time- and temperature-dependent nature of acquired FVIII inhibitors has important implications for the laboratory detection of acquired hemophilia A (see Approach).

EPIDEMIOLOGY

With an incidence estimated to be between 1 and 2 cases per million population per year, acquired hemophilia A is rare disease.[10] The 2012 prospective EACH2 study captured the clinical and demographic characteristics of 501 European patients with acquired hemophilia A, who presented between 2003 and 2008.[11] It showed that the median age at presentation was 73.9 years (range, 61.4–80.4 years), with an even split between males and females. There have been rare reports of acquired hemophilia A in children as young as age 8, and also in the extreme elderly (≥ 85 years).[12,13]

Acquired hemophilia A seems to be caused by a combination of genetic and environmental factors, leading to a breakdown of immune tolerance.[14,15] At this time, it is not possible to predict whether a particular individual will develop a FVIII inhibitor. However, acquired hemophilia A is associated with several underlying conditions.[2] Approximately 10% of acquired hemophilia A is associated with malignancy, with both solid tumors and hematologic malignancies reported. Case series suggest that there is a close temporal relationship between the appearance of the inhibitor and a tumor diagnosis, and that less advanced cancer is associated with inhibitors that

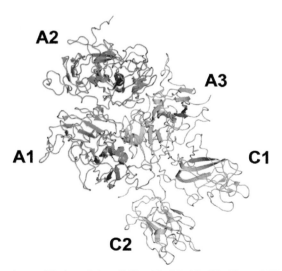

Fig. 1. Tertiary structure of B-domainless FVIII with A1, A2, A3, C1, and C2 domains labeled. By Mattkosloski (21 January 2013), distributed under a CC-BY 3.0 license. Available at: https://en.wikipedia.org/wiki/Factor_VIII#/media/File:Fviii_2R7E.png.

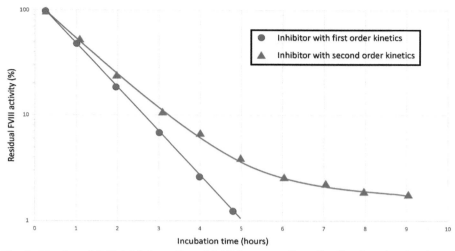

Fig. 2. Kinetics of FVIII inhibitors. Type 1 inhibitors are alloantibodies that develop in patients with congenital hemophilia A, and typically demonstrate first-order (linear) kinetics. Type 2 inhibitors are alloantibodies that develop in patients with acquired hemophilia A, and typically demonstrate second-order (nonlinear) kinetics. These acquired inhibitors rapids neutralize FVIII. However an equilibrium is soon reached, and residual FVIII can be detected in vitro. This residual FVIII activity is not, however, associated with a decreased risk of bleeding in vivo.

are more responsive to treatment.[16] Autoimmune disease underlies approximately another 10% of acquired hemophilia A, with the most common conditions reported to be rheumatoid arthritis and systemic lupus erythematosus.[1,17,18] Pregnancy is an important association in women with acquired hemophilia A, with most inhibitors diagnosed in the puerperium. Women with pregnancy-associated FVIII inhibitors tend to have good clinical outcomes; this is likely due to their young age, generally good health, and the transient nature of their underlying condition.[19] FVIII inhibitors have also been associated with drugs, including antibiotics (penicillin, sulfonamides), immunomodulatory agents (interferon, fludarabine), and antiepileptic drugs (phenytoin).[2] Approximately 50% of cases of acquired hemophilia A are idiopathic, with no underlying cause found.[2]

APPROACH
General Approach to Evaluation

Acquired hemophilia A should be suspected in any bleeding patient with an isolated elevation of the activated partial thromboplastin time (aPTT). Cooperation between the clinician and the laboratory is essential to evaluating the patient and confirming the diagnosis.

Clinical Evaluation

The clinical presentation of acquired hemophilia A is not identical to congenital hemophilia A.[11] Although the latter often manifests as joint bleeding, the former manifests as soft tissue, mucosal, or muscle bleeding. Bleeding in acquired hemophilia A occurs spontaneously, with minimal trauma. Severe bleeding, including gastrointestinal and intracranial bleeds, can also be seen in acquired hemophilia A. Bleeding can be highly morbid in acquired hemophilia A; the 2012 EACH2 survey identified that 87% of patients experienced major bleeding, and 22% died from complications of their inhibitor.[11] Bleeding remains a risk until the FVIII inhibitor has been eliminated.[20] Males and females are also equally affected with acquired hemophilia A, unlike in congenital hemophilia A, where males tend to have more severe bleeding symptoms. And although congenital hemophilia A tends to present in childhood, especially in its moderate and severe forms, acquired hemophilia A tends to manifest in older people.[2]

The clinical evaluation of the patient should focus on establishing the degree and time course of bleeding, as well as the presence of any possible underlying conditions. Clinicians should examine the patient for hematomas; inquire about severe, sustained, or unusual blood loss; and educate the patient about the risk of life- and limb-threatening bleeding. It is vital that clinicians (and patients) note even mild bleeding, so it can be monitored for progression.

Nearly all patients with acquired hemophilia A present with bleeding, and more than 80% of patients with acquired hemophilia A experience hemorrhage or bleeding significant enough to merit transfusion.[1,11,21] Patients with soft tissue bleeding can present with pain, color change, and swelling of the limbs; this condition can easily be confused with deep vein thrombosis and can rapidly progress to compartment syndrome if not managed with hemostatic treatment. The regular monitoring of pain, pulses, sensory function, and motor function is important to ensure soft tissue bleeding does not progress to limb loss. Patients can also develop rapidly evolving intracranial hemorrhages in acquired hemophilia A, so any change in neurologic status should prompt clinical and radiographic assessment. And even minor interventions, such as arterial line placement or venipuncture, can provoke severe bleeding; these procedures should be minimized.

Laboratory Evaluation

Acquired hemophilia A presents a diagnostic challenge, and can easily be confused with other coagulopathies. It should be suspected in any patient with an abnormal aPTT and a normal prothrombin time, international normalized ratio, thrombin time, fibrinogen, and platelet count; however, the differential diagnosis of this finding can also include congenital factor deficiencies, nonspecific inhibitors, and anticoagulants like heparin (**Fig. 3**).

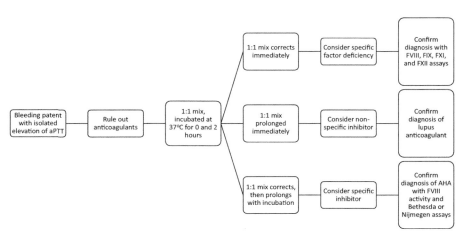

Fig. 3. Laboratory workup of an isolated elevation of aPTT.

The first step in working up an isolated prolongation of the aPTT is determining if the patient is bleeding. Acquired hemophilia A nearly always comes to clinicians' attention because of bleeding (see Clinical Evaluation). Next, heparin contamination of the sample should be ruled out, either by redrawing a blood sample from an uncontaminated peripheral vein, by performing a thrombin time and a reptilase time, or by attempting to neutralize any heparin in the sample with protamine or heparinase. The presence of FXa inhibitors (including low molecular-weight-heparin, fondaparinux, apixaban, rivaroxaban, and edoxaban) can be ruled out with an anti-Xa assay. Once anticoagulants have been ruled out, it is prudent to look back at previous laboratory results for the patient, if available; unlike a congenital factor deficiency (of factors VIII, IX, or XI, or of the so-called intrinsic factors), previous aPTTs should be normal in a patient with acquired hemophilia A.

The use of a 1:1 mix in the diagnostic assessment of acquired coagulation factor inhibitors is controversial. Classical teaching is that when patient plasma is mixed with normal pooled plasma, complete correction of the aPTT suggests a factor deficiency. Conversely, partial or no correction suggests an inhibitor, either specific (eg, FVIII inhibitors) or nonspecific (ie, lupus anticoagulant). Mixing studies are straightforward to perform, even in lower resource settings. They can provide valuable clues to the presence of an underlying inhibitor. However, caution should be exercised when interpreting mixing studies, because they are not standardized and different procedures can lead to different results.[22] The appropriate mixing study to investigate an acquired inhibitor is the 2-step mixing study, which looks at aPTT correction immediately after mixing and then at 1 and 2 hours while the sample is incubated at 37 °C. Samples from patients with acquired hemophilia A may "correct" immediately after mixing. However, the time- and temperature-dependent nature of the acquired FVIII inhibitor is demonstrated by partial or no correction with warming and incubation. A weak inhibitor tends to require a longer incubation ($\geq$2 hours) to demonstrate partial or no correction of the 1:1 mix.[23] It is important for the treating clinician to communicate with their coagulation laboratory when ordering mixing studies, to understand how the assay is performed and reported.

The presence of a lupus anticoagulant can confound or confuse the diagnosis of acquired hemophilia A. A lupus anticoagulant does cause an isolated prolonged aPTT, similar to an acquired FVIII inhibitor[24]; however, it does not cause a bleeding phenotype. Because a lupus anticoagulant causes immediate and sustained inhibition, a 1:1 mixing study will immediately fail to correct—and this result will be sustained despite warming and incubation.[23]

The definitive laboratory tests to diagnose acquired hemophilia A are the FVIII activity and the FVIII inhibitor (Bethesda) assay.[25] FVIII activity is reduced in acquired hemophilia A, but affected individuals often have some detectable FVIII activity in vitro. This occurs because of the inhibitor's second-order kinetics; after a rapid phase, inactivation of FVIII slows to an equilibrium. Yet this residual in vitro activity does not translate into a decreased bleeding risk in vivo.[11,23] The Bethesda assay is used to detect and determine the strength of the FVIII inhibitor. In this assay, serial dilutions of patient plasma are incubated with normal pooled plasma for 2 hours at 37 °C. FVIII activity is then measured at each dilution. The incubated control is considered to be 100% FVIII activity, and the reciprocal dilution of patient plasma that yields 50% FVIII activity is defined as a Bethesda unit (BU).[23,26] For example, if the residual FVIII activity is 50% with a dilution of 1:10, then the actual inhibitor titer within the plasma sample is 10 BU. A stronger inhibitor requires additional dilution to allow FVIII activity to break through, and is thus assigned a higher BU. We consider low-titer inhibitors to be less than 5 BU and high titer inhibitors to be 5 BU or greater.

The classical Bethesda assay can underestimate inhibitor titers at very low titers (<1 BU). This is because changes in pH and protein concentration affect the stability of FVIII inactivation, and these changes can have a large impact on weaker inhibitors. To account for this, some laboratories use a Nijmegen-modified Bethesda assay when the inhibitor titer is low or suspected to be low, buffering the normal plasma and using immunodepleted FVIII deficient plasma to make the serial dilutions.[27–30] Heat treatment of the sample may also improve test sensitivity with low titer inhibitors.[23,28]

THERAPEUTIC OPTIONS

The management of acquired hemophilia A involves 2 parallel strategies: the treatment of bleeding and eradication of the inhibitor.

Treat Bleeding

Clinicians have 2 options for immediate treatment of bleeding in acquired hemophilia A: increasing FVIII levels to overwhelm the inhibitor and bypassing FVIII to activate coagulation despite the presence of the inhibitor. If the bleeding is not severe and the inhibitor titer is less than 5 BU, it is reasonable to attempt local control and focus on increasing plasma FVIII levels. A target of 30% to 50% is generally adequate to achieve hemostasis.[31] Hemostasis can sometimes be achieved with 1-deamino-8-D-arginine vasopressin (DDAVP). DDAVP is a synthetic analogue of the antidiuretic hormone vasopressin, and it increases circulating levels of FVIII.[32] Doses of 0.3 µg/kg subcutaneously daily for 3 to 5 days are typically used in acquired hemophilia A. However, unless the inhibitor titer is very low (<3 BU), DDAVP is often insufficient to manage bleeding.[33]

Severe bleeding with a low titer inhibitor (<5 BU) may be managed with local control and FVIII concentrate, again aiming for a plasma FVIII level of 30% to 50%.[34] Human FVIII replacement is generally not effective, because it is quickly overcome by all but the lowest titer inhibitor. It should be used as a first-line therapy only if no other alternatives are available. Conversely, porcine (pig) FVIII has in vivo activity in humans, but its protein sequence is different enough from human FVIII that it is less affected by acquired FVIII inhibitors. A recombinant porcine FVIII product (OB-1, Obizur) has been shown to control bleeding in acquired hemophilia A, particularly when given as a primary therapy.[35] (All patients in this prospective study also received immunosuppression, and some patients developed inhibitors to Obizur.) The usual starting dose of Obizur is 50 to 100 U/kg. Because incremental recovery is often inadequate, FVIII activity should be checked every 2 to 3 hours, with repeat dosing as needed. It is important to note that patients can develop antiporcine FVIII antibodies in response to the administration of recombinant porcine FVIII; this point limits the effectiveness of subsequent doses, and patients may require a higher initial dose (eg, 200 U/kg) for severe bleeding.

Factor bypassing agents are a more effective way to treat bleeding in acquired hemophilia A, particularly if it is severe and associated with a high titer inhibitor. Both activated prothrombin complex concentrate (aPCC) or recombinant factor VIIa (rFVIIa) have been successfully used in acquired hemophilia A. The EACH2 registry (which was reported before the approval of recombinant porcine FVIII) demonstrated that bleeding was most successfully controlled with bypassing agents with (>90% achieving control), when compared with human FVIII and DDAVP.[33] There was no appreciable difference between rfVIIa and aPCC.

Recombinant FVIIa acts by binding to the surface of activated platelets and promoting thrombin generation directly, independent of FVIII.[36] Studies using rFVIIa as a second-line agent for the treatment of acquired hemophilia A showed a response rate of more than 90% and a complete response rate of 75%.[37] The starting dose of rFVIIa is 70 to 90 μg/kg, repeated every 2 to 3 hours until bleeding stops. The dosing interval can then be lengthened. There is no accurate way to monitor response to rFVIIa treatment with laboratory assays, so clinical monitoring is essential. The most important side effect of rFVIIa is thrombosis—both arterial and venous.[38,39] This complication is most common in older patients, patients with a history of thrombosis, and patients with an underlying prothrombotic condition (eg, cancer).[33]

Activated PCC is a plasma-derived concentrates containing clotting factors II, VII, IX, and X (in both activated and inactivated forms). A retrospective study of aPCC in acquired hemophilia A showed a complete response rate of more than 80% with a dosing regimen of 75 U/kg every 8 to 12 hours until bleeding stopped.[40] (A median number of 10 doses was required to control severe bleeding.) The EACH2 registry demonstrated that 93.3% of bleeds were controlled successfully when aPCC was given.[33] Like rFVIIa, the response to aPCC treatment cannot be monitored accurately with standard laboratory assays, so clinical monitoring is required. In addition, aPCCs carries a risk of thrombosis; daily doses should be limited to less than 200 U/kg to minimize this risk. Because aPCCs contain small amounts of FVIII, they can also trigger an anamnestic increase in inhibitor titer.[26]

Because registry data suggest that both rFVIIa and aPCC are similarly effective, clinicians should use the product that is most available at their center and with which they are most comfortable.

Eradicate the Inhibitor

Surveys of patients with acquired hemophilia A who do not receive immunosuppression suggest that in about one-third of patients, the inhibitor will disappear spontaneously.[41] These spontaneously remitting inhibitors tend to be associated with the postpartum state or with drugs.[1] However, it is not possible to predict at the outset if or when an inhibitor will remit spontaneously. And as long as an acquired FVIII inhibitor persists, there is a risk of serious bleeding. For this reason, most patients undergo immunosuppressive therapy to eradicate their inhibitor.

There are no randomized trial data demonstrating the superiority of any one immunosuppressive regimen, although registry data suggest that combining steroids with additional agents may increase the likelihood of remission.[42] Rituximab-based regimens seem to take longer to effect complete remission. And regardless of the choice of first-line therapy, second-line therapy, if required, can still be successful in approximately 60% of patients.[43]

Corticosteroids are often the first choice for immunosuppression in patients with acquired hemophilia A. Most clinicians are familiar with these drugs, and the risk of serious side effects associated with their short-term use is low. Prednisolone at a dose of 1 mg/kg/d, or prednisone 1 mg/kg/d, eradicates inhibitors in approximately 30% of patients, generally within 3 weeks.[43,44] Adding cyclophosphamide to nonresponding patients at a dose of 2 mg/kg/d can increase the response rate to nearly 70%. It can take up to 6 weeks to demonstrate a response to steroids and cyclophosphamide, and there is a risk of relapse when they are stopped.[43,44]

Second-line therapy for acquired hemophilia A includes inhibitor removal with plasmapheresis or immunoadsorption, azathioprine, vincristine, mycophenolate mofetil, intravenous immunoglobulin, or combined protocols.[45] Because the majority of patients respond to corticosteroids and cyclophosphamide, these agents are not recommended as initial therapy.[45]

Rituximab, an anti-CD20 monoclonal antibody, can be effective in patients who have failed or who cannot tolerate first-line therapy. It seems to confer durable remission in patients with acquired hemophilia A, and most responses occur within the first 2 weeks of therapy.[46–49] Its use in acquired hemophilia A remains off-label in many jurisdictions at this time, but the most commonly used dosing regimen is 375 mg/m^2 weekly for 4 weeks.

Patients receiving immunosuppressive treatment should have FVIII activity levels and inhibitor titers monitored weekly, until the inhibitor becomes undetectable and FVIIII activity goes back to normal.[45]

Focus on Pregnancy

Pregnant women with acquired hemophilia A are managed very similarly to nonpregnant patients. Steroids are the safest and most effective option to eradicate inhibitors.[50] Pregnancy-associated FVIII inhibitors, although they have a lower relapse rate overall, can recur in subsequent pregnancies. Because FVIII inhibitors tend to be IgG antibodies, they can cross the placenta and result in life-threatening fetal and neonatal hemorrhage.[12] For this reason, it is essential to eradicate pregnancy-associated FVIII inhibitors in the first instance and closely monitor patients in subsequent pregnancies.[19]

CLINICAL OUTCOMES

Acquired hemophilia A is a highly morbid condition. Mortality is estimated to range between 15% and 50%, with older patients and those with underlying malignancy at greatest risk of death.[51] The direct cause of death is not always bleeding—patients can die from complications of bleeding, from their underlying disease, or from complications of treatment. The EACH2 registry found that immunosuppressive therapy accounted for 16% of all deaths.[11] This underscores the adverse effects associated with immunosuppression to eradicate inhibitors.

Modern studies suggest that more than 70% of patients achieve complete remission with immunosuppression, which makes it the treatment option of choice. Even when patients relapse after a first complete remission, more than 60% of them go on to achieve a second complete remission.[21,43] Patients with lower titer antibodies and higher residual FVIII activity tend to achieve remission more readily, as do pregnant patients.[52] Patients on immunosuppression generally experience a decrease in inhibitor titer or a risk in baseline FVIII level after 3 to 5 weeks of therapy. If they do not, second-line therapy should be considered. Once remission has been achieved, patients should be monitored for relapse, initially with FVIII activity, and then clinically. EACH2 suggested that relapse occurs in 18% of patients who achieved remission on steroids alone and in 12% receiving corticosteroids and cyclophosphamide, whereas only 3% of patients achieving remission with rituximab-based regimens relapsed. The median time to relapse in this study was approximately 135 days.[43]

Patients receiving treatment should be monitored for adverse effects, including thrombosis from FVIII bypassing agents, and infectious complications of immunosuppression. A UK surveillance study demonstrated that 33% of patients developed sepsis and, in 12% of patients, sepsis contributed to death.[21] Of the patients in the EACH2 registry, 4.2% died from complications of immunosuppression.[43]

DISCUSSION

Further research is needed to improve outcomes for patients with acquired hemophilia A. Novel treatment strategies currently being explored include the use of emicizumab—a recombinant bispecific monoclonal antibody that bridges FIXa and FX, functioning like FVIIIa.[53–56] However, on a more fundamental level, our understanding of which patients respond best to inhibitor eradication treatments and which patients are most likely to attain sustained remission remains incomplete. Future studies of this rare disease should help us to develop better treatment strategies, to help patients achieve durable responses with minimal side effects.

SUMMARY

Acquired hemophilia A is a bleeding disorder caused by antibody formation to FVIII. Acquired hemophilia A manifests as spontaneous, often severe bleeding in individuals with no previous bleeding history. Patients are often older and may have an underlying condition (eg, cancer, autoimmune disorder, pregnancy, drugs). The laboratory manifestations of acquired hemophilia A include an isolated prolongation of the aPTT, decreased FVIII activity, and an inhibitor detectable by the Bethesda assay (with Nijmegen modification for low titer antibodies). Treatment of acquired hemophilia A includes early detection, management of bleeding with hemostatic agents, and eradication of the inhibitor. Acquired hemophilia A is a highly morbid condition; patients suffer the grave effects of bleeding and also of their treatments. Although a majority of patients with acquired hemophilia A will achieve remission—with an undetectable inhibitor titer and cessation of bleeding symptoms—many will die from its complications. Prompt recognition of this bleeding disorder, coupled with evidence-based care, is vital.

CLINICS CARE POINTS

- Acquired hemophilia A should be suspected in any bleeding patient with an isolated elevation of the activated partial thromboplastin time (aPTT).
- Acquired hemophilia A often manifests as soft tissue, mucosal, or muscle bleeding, occurring spontaneously, with minimal trauma. Severe, life threatening bleeding can occur.
- Clinical evaluation should focus on establishing the degree and time course of bleeding, and exploring underlying conditions. 50% of acquired hemophilia A is due to underlying conditions, including pregnancy, autoimmune disease, drugs, or cancer.
- The definitive laboratory tests to diagnose acquired hemophilia A are the FVIII activity and the FVIII inhibitor (Bethesda) assay.
- The management of acquired hemophilia A involves 2 parallel strategies: the treatment of bleeding and eradication of the inhibitor.

DISCLOSURE

The authors have no commercial or financial conflicts of interest.

REFERENCES

1. Green D, Lechner K. A survey of 215 non-hemophilic patients with inhibitors to factor VIII. Thromb Haemost 1981;45(3):200–3.
2. Franchini M, Gandini G, Di Paolantonio T, et al. Acquired hemophilia A: a concise review. Am J Hematol 2005;80(1):55–63.
3. Lavigne-Lissalde G, Schved J-F, Granier C, et al. Anti-factor VIII antibodies: a 2005 update. Thromb Haemost 2005;94(4):760–9.

4. Pratt KP, Shen BW, Takeshima K, et al. Structure of the C2 domain of human factor VIII at 1.5 A resolution. Nature 1999;402(6760):439–42.

5. Prescott R, Nakai H, Saenko EL, et al. The inhibitor antibody response is more complex in hemophilia A patients than in most nonhemophiliacs with factor VIII autoantibodies. Recombinate and Kogenate Study Groups. Blood 1997;89(10): 3663–71.

6. Scandella D, Gilbert GE, Shima M, et al. Some factor VIII inhibitor antibodies recognize a common epitope corresponding to C2 domain amino acids 2248 through 2312, which overlap a phospholipid-binding site. Blood 1995;86(5): 1811–9.

7. Biggs R, Austen DE, Denson KW, et al. The mode of action of antibodies which destroy factor VIII. I. Antibodies which have second-order concentration graphs. Br J Haematol 1972;23(2):125–35.

8. Biggs R, Austen DE, Denson KW, et al. The mode of action of antibodies which destroy factor VIII. II. Antibodies which give complex concentration graphs. Br J Haematol 1972;23(2):137–55.

9. Hoyer LW, Scandella D. Factor VIII inhibitors: structure and function in autoantibody and hemophilia A patients. Semin Hematol 1994;31(2 Suppl 4):1–5.

10. Richter T, Nestler-Parr S, Babela R, et al. Rare disease terminology and definitions—a systematic global review: report of the ISPOR rare disease special interest group. Value Health 2015;18(6):906–14.

11. Knoebl P, Marco P, Baudo F, et al. Demographic and clinical data in acquired hemophilia A: results from the European Acquired Haemophilia Registry (EACH2). J Thromb Haemost 2012;10(4):622–31.

12. Franchini M, Zaffanello M, Lippi G. Acquired hemophilia in pediatrics: a systematic review. Pediatr Blood Cancer 2010;55(4):606–11.

13. Moraca RJ, Ragni MV. Acquired anti-FVIII inhibitors in children. Haemophilia 2002;8(1):28–32.

14. Pavlova A, Zeitler H, Scharrer I, et al. HLA genotype in patients with acquired haemophilia A. Haemophilia 2010;16(102):107–12.

15. Reding MT. Immunological aspects of inhibitor development. Haemophilia 2006; 12(Suppl 6):30–5 [discussion 35–6].

16. Hauser I, Lechner K. Solid tumors and factor VIII antibodies. Thromb Haemost 1999;82(3):1005–7.

17. Green D, Schuette PT, Wallace WH. Factor VIII antibodies in rheumatoid arthritis. Effect of cyclophosphamide. Arch Intern Med 1980;140(9):1232–5.

18. Soriano RM, Matthews JM, Guerado-Parra E. Acquired haemophilia and rheumatoid arthritis. Br J Rheumatol 1987;26(5):381–3.

19. Tengborn L, Baudo F, Huth-Kühne A, et al. Pregnancy-associated acquired haemophilia A: results from the European Acquired Haemophilia (EACH2) registry. BJOG Int J Obstet Gynaecol 2012;119(12):1529–37.

20. Hay CR. Acquired haemophilia. Baillieres Clin Haematol 1998;11(2):287–303.

21. Collins PW, Hirsch S, Baglin TP, et al. Acquired hemophilia A in the United Kingdom: a 2-year national surveillance study by the United Kingdom Haemophilia Centre Doctors' Organisation. Blood 2007;109(5):1870–7.

22. Yates SG, Fitts E, De Simone N, et al. Prolonged partial thromboplastin time: to mix or not to mix – is that the question? Transfus Apher Sci 2019;58(1):39–42.

23. Tiede A, Werwitzke S, Scharf RE. Laboratory diagnosis of acquired hemophilia A: limitations, consequences, and challenges. Semin Thromb Hemost 2014;40(7): 803–11.

24. Devreese KMJ, Ortel TL, Pengo V, et al. Subcommittee on Lupus Anticoagulant/ Antiphospholipid Antibodies. Laboratory criteria for antiphospholipid syndrome: communication from the SSC of the ISTH. J Thromb Haemost JTH 2018;16(4): 809–13.

25. Kasper CK, Aledort L, Aronson D, et al. Proceedings: a more uniform measurement of factor VIII inhibitors. Thromb Diath Haemorrh 1975;34(2):612.

26. Hay CRM, Brown S, Collins PW, et al. The diagnosis and management of factor VIII and IX inhibitors: a guideline from the United Kingdom Haemophilia Centre Doctors Organisation. Br J Haematol 2006;133(6):591–605.

27. Giles AR, Verbruggen B, Rivard GE, et al. A detailed comparison of the performance of the standard versus the Nijmegen modification of the Bethesda assay in detecting factor VIII:C inhibitors in the haemophilia A population of Canada. Association of Hemophilia Centre Directors of Canada. Factor VIII/IX Subcommittee of Scientific and Standardization Committee of International Society on Thrombosis and Haemostasis. Thromb Haemost 1998;79(4):872–5.

28. Batty P, Moore GW, Platton S, et al. Diagnostic accuracy study of a factor VIII ELISA for detection of factor VIII antibodies in congenital and acquired haemophilia A. Thromb Haemost 2015;114(4):804–11.

29. Reber G, Aurousseau MH, Dreyfus M, et al. Inter-laboratory variability of the measurement of low titer factor VIII:C inhibitor in haemophiliacs: improvement by the Nijmegen modification of the Bethesda assay and the use of common lyophilized plasmas. Haemophilia 1999;5(4):292–3.

30. Verbruggen B, Novakova I, Wessels H, et al. The Nijmegen modification of the Bethesda assay for factor VIII:C inhibitors: improved specificity and reliability. Thromb Haemost 1995;73(2):247–51.

31. Gandini G, Franchini M, Manzato F, et al. A combination of prednisone, high-dose intravenous immunoglobulin and desmopressin in the treatment of acquired hemophilia A with high-titer inhibitor. Haematologica 1999;84(11):1054.

32. Franchini M, Lippi G. The use of desmopressin in acquired haemophilia A: a systematic review. Blood Transfus 2011;9(4):377–82.

33. Baudo F, Collins P, Huth-Kühne A, et al. Management of bleeding in acquired hemophilia A: results from the European Acquired Haemophilia (EACH2) Registry. Blood 2012;120(1):39–46.

34. Franchini M, Lippi G. Acquired factor VIII inhibitors. Blood 2008;112(2):250–5.

35. Kruse-Jarres R, St-Louis J, Greist A, et al. Efficacy and safety of OBI-1, an antihaemophilic factor VIII (recombinant), porcine sequence, in subjects with acquired haemophilia A. Haemophilia 2015;21(2):162–70.

36. Hoffman M, Monroe DM, Roberts HR. Platelet-dependent action of high-dose factor VIIa. Blood 2002;100(1):364–5, author reply 365.

37. Hay CR, Negrier C, Ludlam CA. The treatment of bleeding in acquired haemophilia with recombinant factor VIIa: a multicentre study. Thromb Haemost 1997; 78(6):1463–7.

38. Amano K, Seita I, Higasa S, et al. Treatment of acute bleeding in acquired haemophilia A with recombinant activated factor VII: analysis of 10-year Japanese postmarketing surveillance data. Haemophilia 2017;23(1):50–8.

39. Guillet B, Pinganaud C, Proulle V, et al. Myocardial infarction occurring in a case of acquired haemophilia during the treatment course with recombinant activated factor VII. Thromb Haemost 2002;88(4):698–9.

40. Sallah S. Treatment of acquired haemophilia with factor eight inhibitor bypassing activity. Haemophilia 2004;10(2):169–73.

41. Lottenberg R, Kentro TB, Kitchens CS. Acquired hemophilia. A natural history study of 16 patients with factor VIII inhibitors receiving little or no therapy. Arch Intern Med 1987;147(6):1077–81.
42. Collins PW, Percy CL. Advances in the understanding of acquired haemophilia A: implications for clinical practice. Br J Haematol 2010;148(2):183–94.
43. Collins P, Baudo F, Knoebl P, et al. Immunosuppression for acquired hemophilia A: results from the European Acquired Haemophilia Registry (EACH2). Blood 2012;120(1):47–55.
44. Green D, Rademaker AW, Briët E. A prospective, randomized trial of prednisone and cyclophosphamide in the treatment of patients with factor VIII autoantibodies. Thromb Haemost 1993;70(5):753–7.
45. Kruse-Jarres R, Kempton CL, Baudo F, et al. Acquired hemophilia A: updated review of evidence and treatment guidance. Am J Hematol 2017;92(7):695–705.
46. Franchini M, Veneri D, Lippi G, et al. The efficacy of rituximab in the treatment of inhibitor-associated hemostatic disorders. Thromb Haemost 2006;96(2):119–25.
47. Wiestner A, Cho HJ, Asch AS, et al. Rituximab in the treatment of acquired factor VIII inhibitors. Blood 2002;100(9):3426–8.
48. Franchini M. Rituximab in the treatment of adult acquired hemophilia A: a systematic review. Crit Rev Oncol Hematol 2007;63(1):47–52.
49. Field JJ, Fenske TS, Blinder MA. Rituximab for the treatment of patients with very high-titre acquired factor VIII inhibitors refractory to conventional chemotherapy. Haemophilia 2007;13(1):46–50.
50. Hauser I, Schneider B, Lechner K. Post-partum factor VIII inhibitors. A review of the literature with special reference to the value of steroid and immunosuppressive treatment. Thromb Haemost 1995;73(1):1–5.
51. Delgado J, Jimenez-Yuste V, Hernandez-Navarro F, et al. Acquired haemophilia: review and meta-analysis focused on therapy and prognostic factors. Br J Haematol 2003;121(1):21–35.
52. Tiede A, Klamroth R, Scharf RE, et al. Prognostic factors for remission of and survival in acquired hemophilia A (AHA): results from the GTH-AH 01/2010 study. Blood 2015;125(7):1091–7.
53. Croteau SE, Wang M, Wheeler AP. 2021 clinical trials update: Innovations in hemophilia therapy. Am J Hematol 2021;96(1):128–44.
54. Möhnle P, Pekrul I, Spannagl M, et al. Emicizumab in the treatment of acquired haemophilia: a case report. Transfus Med Hemother 2019;46(2):121–3.
55. Al-Banaa K, Alhillan A, Hawa F, et al. Emicizumab use in treatment of acquired hemophilia a: a case report. Am J Case Rep 2019;20:1046–8.
56. Dane KE, Lindsley JP, Streiff MB, et al. Successful use of emicizumab in a patient with refractory acquired hemophilia A and acute coronary syndrome requiring percutaneous coronary intervention. Res Pract Thromb Haemost 2019;3(3):420–3.

Hemophilia B (Factor IX Deficiency)

Robert F. Sidonio Jr, MD, MSc[a],*, Lynn Malec, MD, MSc[b]

KEYWORDS

- Hemophilia B • Factor IX • Prophylaxis • Treatment • Extravascular distribution

KEY POINTS

- With an incidence of approximately 5 cases per 100,000 individuals, hemophilia B is rarer than hemophilia A and has important differences related to the genetic mutations, bleeding severity, rates of inhibitor development, and eradication.
- Factor IX has unique physiologic properties as compared with factor VIII, including its large extravascular distribution, which accounts for approximately 70% of total body factor IX.
- The mainstay of hemophilia B therapy for those with severe phenotypic disease is prophylactic administration of factor IX replacement therapy; recent advances in half-life extension for FIX products allow for an approximately 60% reduction in annualized doses of FIX required for prophylaxis.
- Ongoing clinical investigation in subcutaneous FIX, novel nonfactor therapies, and gene therapy/editing is underway and may further advance the available treatment options for those living with hemophilia B.

INTRODUCTION

Hemophilia B is a rare congenital bleeding disorder owing to a deficiency of coagulation factor IX (FIX). It is an X-linked disorder that results from pathogenic variants in the *F9* gene and is seen in all racial and ethnic populations. As compared with hemophilia A (a deficiency of coagulation factor VIII [FVIII]), hemophilia B is much less common and estimated to account for 15% to 20% of all hemophilia cases.[1] Although similar, there are important aspects of FIX biology and hemophilia B treatment that should be considered for optimal management of affected individuals (**Fig. 1**).

History

Historically, hemophilia A and hemophilia B were thought to be the same disorder until 1947 when decreased FVIII levels were described with hemophilia A.[2] Five years later

[a] Emory University, 1760 Haygood Drive, HSRB W340, Atlanta, GA 30322, USA; [b] Versiti Blood Research Institute, 8733 Watertown Plank Road, Milwaukee, WI 53213, USA
* Corresponding author.
E-mail address: robert.sidonio.jr@emory.edu

Hematol Oncol Clin N Am 35 (2021) 1143–1155
https://doi.org/10.1016/j.hoc.2021.07.008
0889-8588/21/© 2021 Elsevier Inc. All rights reserved.

Differences Between Hemophilia A and Hemophilia B

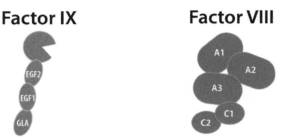

Factor IX   ## Factor VIII

	Hemophilia B	Hemophilia A
Prevalence	1 in 30 000 males	1 in 5 000 males
Inheritance	X-linked recessive (F9;Xq27)	X-linked recessive (F8; Xq28)
Molecular characteristics	----------------------	----------------------
Hemostatic function	Enzyme	Co-factor
Size/structure	55 kDa (34kb; 8 exons)	280 kDa (180kb; 26 exons)
Half-life (wild type)	18–24h	12–14h
Concentration in plasma	3–5 µg/mL	0.1–0.25 µg/mL
Genetic variants	Missense variants in >60% of SHB	Null variants in >80% of SHA
Cross reactive material (CRM)+	~55%	~5%
Inhibitor development	----------------------	----------------------
Risk (severe, non-severe)	4–5%, ~0%	30–40%, 5–10%
Complications	Hypersensitivity (>60%), bleeding, nephrotic syndrome	Well tolerated, bleeding
Success	~20–30%	60–70%

Fig. 1. Highlights of the difference between hemophilia A and hemophilia B. FVIII or F8, factor VIII; FIX or F9, factor IX.

in 1952, hemophilia B was recognized as a distinct entity when the first patient, Stephen Christmas, was described in the literature, giving rise to the eponym "Christmas disease" for hemophilia B.[3] These early discoveries paved the way for the modern era of hemophilia treatment with the discovery of plasma fractions containing factor IX in the 1960s.[4] In the recent decades, hemophilia therapy has continued to rapidly evolve, including approval of recombinant extended half-life (EHL) products now used by most patients with severe hemophilia B in the United States who receive prophylaxis.[5] Additional novel nonfactor therapies targeting inhibitors of coagulation and gene therapy are in clinical development and will likely provide additional treatment options for patients to further allow for personalization of therapy in hemophilia B in the coming decades.

DISCUSSION
Biology of Factor IX in Hemostasis

Factor IX is a vitamin K–dependent enzyme that is essential for normal thrombin generation. It is synthesized in the liver as a polypeptide with notable posttranslational modifications including but not limited to γ-carboxylation, partial β-hydroxylation, O- and N-glycosylation, and sulfation and phosphorylation.[6] The circulating zymogen

FIX undergoes activation by release of the activation peptide. The 2 principal activators of the zymogen are activated factor IX (IXa) and the tissue factor:activated factor VII complex. IXa complexes with activated factor VIII, calcium, and phosphatidylserine to generate activated factor X (Xa), which forms the prothrombinase complex. The prothrombinase complex, consisting of factor Xa, activated factor V, and calcium, is essential for the conversion of prothrombin to thrombin, which is crucial in regulation of hemostasis. Thrombin in turn is essential for fibrin generation, clot retraction, and activation of factor XIII. The decrease or absence of factor IX as seen in hemophilia B impairs the generation of thrombin and fibrin, which results in hemorrhage with minimal (or unknown) trauma and potentially life-threatening bleeding.

Extravascular distribution of factor IX

In contrast to FVIII, which circulates and remains in the bloodstream in complex with von Willebrand factor, FIX has significant distribution outside of the intravascular compartment. Factor IX can be detected in the vascular wall,[7–9] where it colocalizes with type IV collagen, a major component of the subendothelial basement membrane (**Fig. 2**). FIX binding to type IV collagen has been shown to be essential for hemostasis, and this subendothelial FIX is important in controlling microbleeding.[10] Stafford's research group argues that localization of FIX near the basement membrane protects it from premature clearance and optimally positions it near the site of vessel injury. Preclinical data suggest that FIX leaves the plasma circulation to bind to type IV collagen within the endothelial matrix, and this extravascular FIX supports hemostasis regardless of the measurable plasma FIX level.[8] Furthermore, the extravascular pool of FIX is in excess of 3-fold higher than the plasma pool, and this remains in a dynamic equilibrium.[10] In 1996, Cheung and colleagues[7] demonstrated that FIX binds to collagen type IV within the endothelial matrix, further supporting liver and muscle histology studies.[9] Interestingly, when the FIX plasma level is at 1%, there is at least 17-fold higher extravascular FIX available.[7] This discrepancy could explain the reduced in vivo recovery and 20% to 40% FIX plasma "loss" to the extravascular space within minutes of exogenous FIX infusion.[11] The functional role of extravascular FIX has been

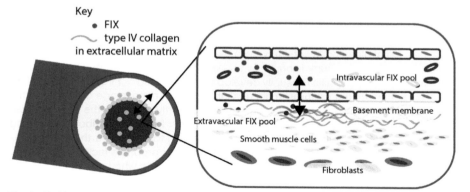

Extravascular Distribution of Factor IX

Key
- FIX
- type IV collagen in extracellular matrix

Intravascular FIX pool
Basement membrane
Extravascular FIX pool
Smooth muscle cells
Fibroblasts

Fig. 2. (*left*) A cross-section of a blood vessel with FIX in the plasma in dynamic equilibrium with the FIX in the extravascular space. (*right*) The movement of FIX. Immediately after infusion, FIX moves from the intravascular to the extravascular space and binds to collagen type IV on the basement membrane within the extracellular matrix.

thoroughly supported by preclinical models demonstrating hemostatic protection arising from this FIX depot despite no apparent measurable plasma FIX.[12,13]

Prevalence of Hemophilia B

The estimated prevalence of hemophilia B is 5 cases per 100,000 male births for all severities of hemophilia B as compared with 24.6 cases for all severities of hemophilia A[14] (see **Fig. 1**). In addition, severe hemophilia B, characterized by an FIX activity of less than 1%, is much less common than severe hemophilia A, with an estimated prevalence of 1.5 cases per 100,000 male births as compared with 9.5 cases with severe hemophilia A.

Transmission of hemophilia

Female carriers of hemophilia can transmit the disorder, causing variant to half of male children who will be affected with hemophilia, and half of female children who will similarly be hemophilia carriers or heterozygotes. The prevalence of sporadic hemophilia in which a male infant is born to a noncarrier mother is encountered in approximately 40% of cases of severe hemophilia B, and 30% of mild and moderate cases.[15] There are likely ∼2 to 3 carriers for every male child born with this X-linked recessive disorder. Assuming ∼100 male children with hemophilia B were born per year, the authors anticipate at least 270 hemophilia B carriers are born per year in the United States. Because of lyonization or skewing, up to 30% of these heterozygous women will have FIX levels less than 40%. In the United States, up to 25% of all affected patients with mild hemophilia B is a woman or girl skewing much more rarely (<2%) to moderate/severe hemophilia B.[16] The bleeding phenotype of male children and female children with the same factor deficiency has not been fully investigated, but treatment should be based on the deficiency and not gender.

Severity of Hemophilia and Clinical Manifestations of Bleeding

Clinically apparent bleeding in hemophilia B typically correlates with the factor IX activity in plasma. Hemophilia B is classified based on this plasma activity as "severe" when FIX levels are less than 0.01 IU/mL, "moderate" when FIX levels are 0.01 to 0.05 IU/mL, and "mild" when FIX levels are greater than 0.05 to 0.40 IU/mL. Clinically evident bleeding typically corresponds to the level of circulating FIX (**Table 1**), although some patients may have variability in phenotypic bleeding with up to 10% of severe patients with a mild phenotype.

- *Severe hemophilia B* (FIX <0.01 IU/mL): In patients with severe hemophilia, bleeding occurs frequently and spontaneously into joints, muscles, and soft tissues. Initial bleeding events may be in the neonatal period related to birth trauma or at the time of circumcision, or by an average age of 10.5 months when infants with severe hemophilia B usually develop their first bleed.[17] First-time bleeds into the joint space (hemarthrosis) occur slightly later at a mean age of 14.2 months. As with hemophilia A, joint bleeding most frequently occurs in the "index joints" of patients with hemophilia, which are the ankles, knees, and elbows. Bleeding occurs throughout the age spectrum and can lead to crippling arthropathy if patients have poor bleed prevention plans or lack of appropriate factor prophylaxis.
- *Moderate hemophilia B* (FIX 0.01–0.05 IU/mL): Patients who have moderate hemophilia B have a more varied bleeding phenotype ranging from almost no spontaneous or minor trauma-related bleeding to severe muscle and joint bleeding as would be seen in severe hemophilia. Joint bleeds and muscle hematomas may occur after mild injury and in some cases may occur without obvious provocation. In those with a more severe phenotypic bleeding pattern, the World

Table 1
Classification of hemophilia B and general treatment recommendations

Classification of Hemophilia	Baseline FIX Activity	Bleeding Manifestations	Treatment Recommendations
Severe	0.01 IU/mL (<1%)	Frequent spontaneous joint & muscle hemorrhages; life-threatening bleeds	Prophylaxis
Moderate	>0.01–0.05 IU/mL (>1%–5%)	Occasional spontaneous joint and muscle hemorrhages; hemorrhage with trauma/surgery	On demand; prophylaxis if phenotypically severe
Mild	>0.05–40 IU/mL (>5%–40%)	Rare spontaneous or minimally traumatic	
Hemorrhage	On demand (rare use of prophylaxis)		

Federation of Hemophilia (WFH) recommends the use of prophylaxis regardless of their baseline FIX activity.

- *Mild hemophilia A* (FIX >0.05–40 IU/mL): In those with mild disease, bleeding typically occurs only with surgery, invasive procedures, or major injury. Given this, some individuals with mild hemophilia may not be diagnosed until late childhood or adulthood. There is debate on the upper limit of "normal" FIX with some using 50% over the traditional 40% FIX level cutoff.

Phenotypic bleeding in hemophilia A as compared with hemophilia B

Although the anatomic locations of bleeding hemophilia overlap, several studies have reported possible differences in bleeding severity in hemophilia B with less severe phenotypic manifestations as compared with hemophilia A. This reduced bleeding tendency could be attributed to the underlying genetic variants in hemophilia B, which tend to be non-null, thus producing some defective FIX, allowing some hemostatic protection. Several early clinical studies demonstrated the likely milder bleeding phenotype of severe hemophilia B compared with severe hemophilia A as evidenced by a smaller proportion of severe hemophilia B requiring factor prophylaxis, lower composite Hemophilia Severity Scores, lower orthopedic joint scores and radiologic joint damage scores, and lower odds of needing arthroplasty. There is likely bias and several conflicting studies as well as inclusion of less than 2% as a previous definition of severe hemophilia B. In summary, the clinician should closely consider observing the bleeding tendency of the individual patient and consider early prophylaxis following evidence of life-threatening or joint bleeding.[18–20]

Genetics of Hemophilia B

The *F9* gene is located near the terminus of the long arm of the X chromosome, is considerably smaller than the *F8* gene at approximately 34 kb in length, and is relatively structurally simple with only 8 exons[21] (see **Fig. 1**). Disease-causing mutations in *F9* are highly heterogeneous and are well studied, with more than 1000 mutations described in relevant databases. Classes of mutations, including point mutations, deletions, insertions, and rearrangements/inversions, have been found in *F9* and *F8*;

however, the relative frequency of these mutations differs by hemophilia type with approximately 60% of severe hemophilia B arising from missense mutations. Mutation types in *F8* and *F9* genes correlate with residual plasma factor activity and bleeding phenotype, with larger gene defects typically associated with a more severe phenotype and higher risk of inhibitor development.

Cross-reactive material and genetic mutation

Cross-reactive material (CRM) is a protein that lacks biological activity but has antigenic determinants in common with normal, hemostatically functional FIX. Given patients with severe hemophilia B are less often to have a null mutation associated with their bleeding disorder, the presence of cross-reactive material (CRM+) influences pharmacokinetic measurements such as in vivo recovery of FIX[9] and may ultimately influence the efficacy of prophylaxis because of competition of defective endogenous FIX for the collagen type IV binding sites from exogenously infused FIX.[10] Because most severe hemophilia B patients are CRM+ compared with severe hemophilia A (<5%), there is a reduced tendency to develop a neutralizing antibody (see **Fig. 1**).

Hemophilia B Leyden

A rare but interesting mutation in the promoter region of the *F9* gene results in an entity known as hemophilia B Leyden.[22] Individuals with hemophilia B Leyden have low FIX levels as children and more severe phenotypic disease; however, because of the mutation in the promoter region being receptive to androgen stimulation, male patients have considerable improvement in FIX levels and disease severity after puberty, and similar improvement is seen during pregnancy in female carriers.

Principles of Hemophilia B Treatment

The overall goal of hemophilia B treatment involves utilization of exogenous clotting factor concentrates, or other novel therapies (not currently approved), to achieve hemostasis. Treatment is aimed at preventing potentially debilitating recurrent joint bleeding leading to joint destruction, known as hemophilic arthropathy, and to provide effective hemostatic control in the event of bleeding events or invasive procedures (**Table 2**). In order to effectively manage bleeding events, knowledge of the baseline factor level, severity and location of hemorrhage, and the presence of anti-factor IX inhibitory antibodies is essential. Delivery of care is best provided through dedicated diagnostic and treatment centers with standardized treatment protocols, ideally at a hemophilia treatment center or hemophilia comprehensive care center[1] guided by a multidisciplinary team.

Acute/critical care for bleeding events

Patients with hemophilia should receive immediate care for potential bleeding events with strong consideration of treatment with clotting factor concentrates before any imaging including, but not limited to, cranial or abdominal imaging. Emergency treatment plans should be in place for basic management to guide emergency room providers for time-sensitive major bleeding events. Bleeding events in the joints (hemarthrosis) or muscles (hematomas) are common in the emergency room setting and warrant immediate care to limit the long-term effects on bone and joint health and avoidance or nerve injury.

Prophylaxis versus on-demand/episodic therapy

Prophylaxis historically involves the routine administration of factor IX concentrate to maintain at least a 1% trough FIX activity in between dosing. Historically, this was done based on the observation that those patients with moderate hemophilia (ie,

FIX activity 1% to 5%) had rare spontaneous bleeding events, but with advances in therapy, higher trough values (3%–5% or higher) may be targeted.[1] Individuals who do not use a regimen of prophylaxis treat at the time of bleeding events, known as treating "on demand" or use "episodic therapy." Much of this data is supported by hemophilia A studies, and the hemostatic role of extravascular FIX (unmeasurable) has questioned this practice in hemophilia B. Until there are clear clinical studies, it is still recommended to target a trough of at least 1%. Determination of how much improved hemostatic protection is conveyed with lower (1%–3%) and higher (15%–30%) trough levels with certain EHL products is under investigation.

Initiation of prophylaxis. Prophylaxis is considered standard of care in all patients with severe hemophilia B, which historically has been defined by factor IX activity (<1%) but more recently has been recommended by the WFH to be used in all patients with phenotypically severe hemophilia regardless of endogenous factor activity.[1] Dosing intensity depends on local resources and availability of clotting factor concentrate. For standard half-life (SHL) FIX products, starting dosing ranges from 15 IU/kg/dose twice a week to 40 to 60 IU/kg/dose twice a week, ideally infused in the morning or before strenuous physical activity.[1] For EHL products, one should follow the label indication as a starting point and then escalate as needed to prevent bleeding.

- For children, according to the Medical and Scientific Advisory Council of the National Hemophilia Foundation,[23] prophylaxis should begin early in life before the onset of recurrent bleeding. WFH similarly recommends initiation of prophylaxis (primary prophylaxis) before the onset of a second hemarthrosis, before evidence of joint damage, and before the age of 3 years.
- For teenagers and adults who may not have previously used prophylaxis, including those that have existing joint damage, prophylaxis should still be offered in order to prevent progression of joint disease.

Factor Replacement and FIX Pharmacokinetics

Factor IX half-life
Factor IX concentrates (plasma derived and SHL recombinant products) have a half-life that is approximately 18 to 24 hours (**Table 3**). Substantial prolongation of half-life

---

Table 2
General treatment recommendation for hemophilia B

Bleed Type	Target Level (%)	Treatment Duration (d)
Joint bleed	50–100	1–2
Intracranial bleed	80–100 (initial)	7
	30–50 (maintenance)	8–21
Small muscle bleed	50	2–3
Deep muscle bleed	80–100 (initial)	1–2
	50 (maintenance)	3–5
Gastrointestinal bleeding	80–100	7–14
Minor surgery	60–80 (preoperatively)	—
	40–50 (maintenance)	1–5
Major surgery	80–100 (preoperatively)	—
	50 (maintenance)	1–14

Table 3
Widely available clotting factor concentrates for treatment of hemophilia B

	Standard Half-Life Recombinant Factor IX Products		
	BeneFIX	Rixubis	Ixinity
Host Cell Label Indication	CHO prophylaxis, surgery, and on-demand bleed control	CHO prophylaxis, surgery, and on-demand bleed control	CHO prophylaxis, surgery, and on-demand bleed control
Available vial sizes (IU)	250 500 1000 2000 3000	250 500 1000 2000 3000	250 500 1000 1500 2000 3000
Technology	N/A	N/A	N/A
Dosing calculation	1.2–1.4 IU/kg raises plasma level by 1%	1.1–1.3 IU/kg raises plasma level by 1%	1 IU/kg raises plasma level by 1%
Half-life, h	14–28	16–27	17–31

	Extended Half-Life Recombinant Factor IX Products		
	Alprolix	Idelvion	Rebinyn
Host Cell Label Indication	HEK prophylaxis, surgery and on demand bleed control	CHO prophylaxis, surgery and on demand bleed control	CHO surgery and on demand bleed control
Available vial sizes (IU)	500 1000 2000 3000	250 500 1000 2000	500 1000 2000
Technology	Fusion of FIX to the dimeric Fc domain of IgG	Fusion of FIX via cleavable linker to albumin	Fusion of FIX to 40 kDa PEG moiety
Dosing calculation	1–1.4 IU/kg raises plasma level by 1%	0.7–1 IU/kg raises plasma level by 1%	1 IU/kg raises plasma level by 1.5%–2.3%
Half-life, h	66.4–86.52	90–104	69.6–89.4

Abbreviations: CHO, Chinese hamster ovary; HEK, human embryonic kidney; N/A, not applicable.

has been achieved through modification of recombinant factor IX therapies (rFIX) through pegylation, albumin fusion, and fusion to the Fc portion of IgG (**Fig. 3**). These modifications have led to a 4- to 6-fold prolongation of the half-life (see **Table 3**). Utilization of EHL-FIX products is estimated to reduce the annual number of infusions needed for prophylaxis by approximately 60%.[24]

Factor IX recovery
The amount of factor IX concentrate that is required to achieve a similar plasma level is approximately twice that of an FVIII product. Generally, each unit of plasma-derived FIX infused per kilogram of body weight will raise the FIX activity by approximately 1 IU/dL, but this varies by age (poorer incremental recovery) and by product type. The recovery of unmodified rFIX is lower, such that each unit of rFIX will raise FIX activity by approximately 0.8 IU/dL in adults and 0.7 IU/dL in children under 15 years of age. Recovery estimations for specific factor therapies may differ, and evaluation of traditional pharmacokinetics or through the use of population models is strongly encouraged (see **Table 3**).

Volume of distribution of factor IX
Because factor IX distributes outside of the vascular space, it has a volume of distribution (VOD) that is distinct from FVIII, which largely remains within the intravascular space (see **Fig. 2**). The pharmacokinetics of FIX is more complex than FVIII and can best be described by a 3-compartment model, including the central compartment (plasma) and peripheral compartments (eg, a protein binding compartment and extracellular space) and may be different depending on modifications in rFIX products[25] (**Fig. 4**). The clinical significance of VOD related to bleed protection and control is not clear but it affects in vivo recovery and dosing.

Complications of Factor Replacement

Inhibitor development
The incidence of alloantibody formation to infused factor concentrates is substantially lower in hemophilia B than in hemophilia A. Approximately 4% to 5% of patients with severe hemophilia B will develop inhibitory antibodies compared with 30% to 40% of severe hemophilia A patients.[26–28] Development of inhibitory antibodies renders factor IX concentrates ineffective and necessitates the utilization of bypassing products to manage bleeding events. Inhibitors to factor IX are primarily seen in the severe subgroup of patients with large gene deletions and nonsense mutations in *F9*.

- Immune tolerance induction (ITI) is an approach to inhibitor eradication through the repeated and frequent administration of FIX (or FVIII in hemophilia A) in an attempt to downregulate the antibody response to FIX. Unfortunately, ITI is less successful (20%–30%) in hemophilia B. Although there is no standardized protocol for ITI in hemophilia B, utilization of a combination of FIX and immunosuppressive agents may be considered first-line therapy in addition to consideration of EHL-FIX products.[29,30]
- Patients with inhibitors can also develop a range from mild hypersensitivity to a severe allergic reaction or anaphylaxis; therefore, if feasible, one should consider a desensitization protocol with administration of incrementally higher doses of FIX concentrates in a critical care/hospital setting.

Recent Innovations in Hemophilia B Therapy

There continues to be ongoing advances in the development of therapeutics to treat hemophilia B. Current studies are underway in the areas of (1) subcutaneous FIX

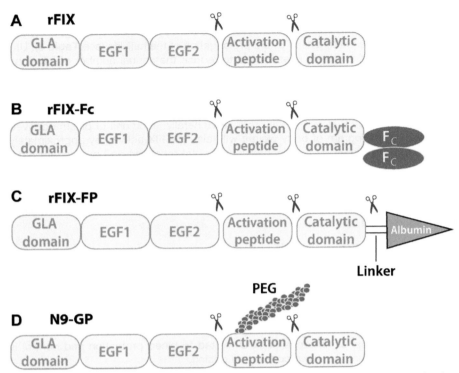

Fig. 3. (A) Wild type rFIX consists of the GLA domain, EGF-1 and EG-2 domains, an activation peptide, and a catalytic domain. The zymogen FIX undergoes proteolytic cleavage and release of the activation peptide. (B) rFIX-Fc is created by binding the Fc domain of IgG1 to the C-terminus extending the half-life of rFIX. (C) rFIX-FP is created by binding albumin via a cleavable linker extending the half-life of rFIX. (D) N9-GP is created by chemically modifying the activation peptide with a site specific 40-kDa PEG molecule. EGF, epidermal growth factor; GLA, gamma-carboxylation; PEG, polyethylene glycol.

products, which aim to lessen the burden of current IV administration of products; (2) nonfactor/novel therapeutics that aim to rebalance the coagulation system; and (3) gene therapy/gene editing, which aims to increase endogenous FIX production and mitigate the need for routine prophylactic factor administration.

Subcutaneous FIX products
Although utilization of EHL-FIX products has reduced the burden of administration and allowed for dosing as infrequently as every 14 to 21 days, there remains a desire to further lessen the treatment intensity through development of subcutaneous products. This could eliminate the need for central venous access or venipuncture training particularly in children; 2 current therapeutics are being investigated, including BIVV002 and dalcinonacog alfa.

Nonfactor/novel therapies
Approaches to "rebalancing" the coagulation system through manipulation of procoagulant and anticoagulant proteins are currently in preclinical and clinical trials. Antithrombin, tissue pathway factor inhibitor, protein C, and protein S have been targeted as novel therapeutic agents. These therapies may offer novel therapies to

Extravasation potentials of various rFIX products

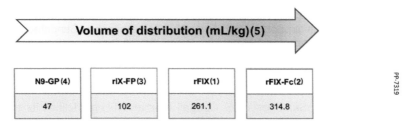

Volume of distribution (mL/kg)(5)

N9-GP(4)	rIX-FP(3)	rFIX(1)	rFIX-Fc(2)
47	102	261.1	314.8

PP-7319

Fig. 4. VOD of the various widely available FIX products. VOD does not imply lack of hemostatic ability, but it may limit the movement of rFIX into the extravascular space. N9-GP, nonacog beta pegol. 1. Benefix Package insert downloaded Jan 2021. 2. ALPROLIX Package insert downloaded Jan 2021. 3. Idelvion Package insert downloaded Jan 2021. 4. Rebinyn package insert downloaded Jan 2021. 5. Iorio A et al. *Thromb Haemost* 2017. The pK of rFIXFc and rFIX is best described by a three compartment model while N9-GP and rFIX-FP is described by a one-compartment model.

patients with hemophilia B with inhibitors who otherwise have poor therapeutic options for prophylaxis. Specific information regarding the safety and efficacy of the medications, including with management of breakthrough bleeding events and surgeries, will require ongoing data from the pivotal clinical trials.

Gene therapy

Over the last approximately 2 decades, preclinical and clinical studies on adeno-associated viral (AAV) vector-based gene therapy for hemophilia have identified successful strategies. Current AAV vector therapy typically uses a transgene under the control of a liver-specific promoter, thus allowing for hepatic tropism and delivery via a single intravenous peripheral injection. Several clinical trials are ongoing in the hemophilia B patient population; however, there is currently no approved gene therapy product in the United States, Europe, or elsewhere. Most platforms are now using the FIX-Padua variant, which confers approximately 8-fold higher activity for equivalent protein expression achieved with wild-type *F9*. A major question in gene therapy is not only the safety (oncologic potential) and tolerability of vector infusion but also the long-term stability of FIX production.[31,32]

CLINICS CARE POINTS

- Prophylaxis should be considered early in life when feasible and prior to recurrent joint bleeding or following a significant bleeding event.

- The clinical significance of volume of distribution related to bleed protection and control is not clear but it affects in vivo recovery and dosing.

- When choosing a FIX product consider the safety track record, inherent pK properties and clinical trial outcomes data (phase III and IV data) to ensure achieving the endpoints that matter to the patient and provider. This includes improved quality of life, confidence in protection and prevention and controlling of bleeding events.

DISCLOSURE

L. Malec has received research support from Sanofi Genzyme. She has received consultancy fees from Bayer, CSL, Sanofi Genzyme, Spark, Takeda, Sobi. R. Sidonio has received research support from Takeda/Shire, Octapharma, Genentech, and Grifols. He has received consultancy fees from Bayer, Sanofi Genzyme, Takeda, Sobi, Spark, Biomarin, Novo Nordisk, Pfizer, and Emergent Solutions.

REFERENCES

1. Srivastava A, Santagostino E, Dougall A, et al. WFH guidelines for the management of hemophilia panelists and co-authors. WFH guidelines for the management of hemophilia, 3rd edition. Haemophilia 2020;26(Suppl 6):1–158.
2. Brinkhous KM. Clotting defect in hemophilia: deficiency in plasma factor required for platelet utilization. Proc Soc Exp Biol Med 1947;66:117–20.
3. Biggs R, Couglas AS, MacFarlane RG, et al. Christmas disease: a condition previous mistake for haemophilia. Br Med J 1952;2:137801382.
4. Tullis JL, Melin M, Jurigian P. Clinical use of human prothrombin complexes. N Engl J Med 1965;273:667–74.
5. Malec LM, Cheng D, Witmer CM, et al. The impact of extended half-life factor concentrates on prophylaxis for severe hemophilia in the United States. Am J Hematol 2020;95(8):960–5.
6. Larson PJ, High KA. Biology of inherited coagulopathies: factor IX. Hematol Oncol Clin North Am 1992;6(5):999–1009.
7. Cheung WF, van den Born J, Kuhn K, et al. Identification of the endothelial cell binding site for factor IX. Proc Natl Acad Sci U S A 1996;93:11068–73.
8. Gui T, Lin HF, Jin DY, et al. Circulating and binding characteristics of wild-type factor IX and certain Gla domain mutants in vivo. Blood 2002;100:153–8.
9. Cooley B, Funkhouser W, Monroe D, et al. Prophylactic efficacy of BeneFIX vs Alprolix in hemophilia B mice. Blood 2016;128:286–92.
10. Stafford DW. Extravascular FIX and coagulation. Thromb J 2016;14(Suppl 1):35.
11. Poon MC, Lillicrap D, Hensman C, et al. Recombinant factor IX recovery and inhibitor safety: a Canadian post-licensure surveillance study. Thromb Haemost 2002;87:431–5, 14.
12. Gui T, Reheman A, Ni H, et al. Abnormal hemostasis in a knock-in mouse carrying a variant of factor IX with impaired binding to collagen type IV. J Thromb Haemost 2009;7:1843–51.
13. Matino D, Iorio A, Stafford D, et al. Enhanced FIX collagen IV binding shows improved hemostatic effects in a hemophilia B mouse model. Top abstract presentation, ISTH SSC Meeting. Dublin, July 18, 2018.
14. Iorio A, Stonebraker JS, Chambost H, et al. Establishing the prevalence and prevalence at birth of hemophilia in males: a metaanalytic approach using national registries. Ann Intern Med 2019;171(8):540–6.
15. Kasper CK, Lin JCSO. Prevalence of sporadic and familial haemophilia 2007;13(1):90.
16. Miller CH, Bean CJ. Genetic causes of haemophilia in women and girls. Haemophilia 2020;27(2):e164–79.
17. Nijdam A, Altisent C, Carcao MD, et al. Bleeding before prophylaxis in severe hemophilia: paradigm shift over two decades. Haematologica 2015;100(3):e84–6.
18. Ludlam CA, Lee RJ, Prescott RJ, et al. Haemophilia care in central Scotland 1980-94. I. Demographic characteristics, hospital admissions and causes of death. Haemophilia 2000;6(5):494–503.

19. Schulman S, Eelde A, Holmström M, et al. Validation of a composite score for clinical severity of hemophilia. J Thromb Haemost 2008;6(7):1113–21.
20. Santagostino E, Mancuso ME, Tripodi A, et al. Severe hemophilia with mild bleeding phenotype: molecular characterization and global coagulation profile. J Thromb Haemost 2010;8(4):737–43.
21. Castaman G, Matino D. Hemophilia A and B: molecular and clinical similarities and differences. Haematologica 2019;104(9):1702–9.
22. Royle G, Van de Water NS, Berry E, et al. Leyden arising de novo by point mutation in the putative factor IX promoter region. Br J Haematol 1991;77(2):191–4.
23. MASAC Document 241. National hemophilia foundation. Available at: https://www.hemophilia.org/healthcare-professionals/guidelines-on-care/masac-documents. Accessed August 31, 2021.
24. Mannucci PM. Hemophilia therapy: the future has begun. Haematologica 2020; 105(3):545–53.
25. Iorio A, Fischer K, Blanchette V. Tailoring treatment of haemophilia B: accounting for the distribution and clearance of standard and extended half-life FIX concentrates. Thromb Haemost 2017;117(06):1023–30.
26. DiMichele D. Inhibitor development in haemophilia B: an orphan disease in need of attention. Br J Haematol 2007;138(3):305–15.
27. Male C, Andersson NG, Rafowicz A, et al. Inhibitor incidence in an unselected cohort of previously untreated patients with severe haemophilia B: a PedNet study. Haematologica 2020;106(1):123–9.
28. Pierce GF, Kaczmarek R, Noone D, et al. Gene therapy to cure haemophilia: is robust scientific inquiry the missing factor? Haemophilia 2020;26(6):931–3.
29. Beutel K, Hauch H, Rischewski J, et al. ITI with high-dose FIX and combined immunosuppressive therapy in a patient with severe haemophilia B and inhibitor. Hamostaseologie 2009;29(2):155–7.
30. Malec L, Abshire T, Jobe S, et al. rFIXFc for immune tolerance induction in a severe hemophilia B patient with an inhibitor and prior history of ITI related nephrotic syndrome. Haemophilia 2018;24(4):e294–6.
31. Nathwani AC, Tuddenham EGD, Rangarajan S, et al. Adenovirus-associated virus vector-mediated gene transfer in hemophilia B. N Engl J Med 2011;365:2357–65.
32. George LA, Sullivan SK, Giermasz A, et al. Hemophilia B gene therapy with a high-specific-activity factor IX variant. N Engl J Med 2017;377(23):2215–27.

Factor XI Deficiency

Magdalena Dorota Lewandowska, MD[a,*], Jean Marie Connors, MD[b]

KEYWORDS

- Factor XI deficiency • Hemophilia C • Rosenthal syndrome
- Plasma thromboplastin antecedent deficiency

KEY POINTS

- FXI deficiency (Hemophilia C or Rosenthal's disease) is distinguished from FVIII and IX deficiency by its autosomal, as opposed to X-linked, inheritance pattern and variable bleeding tendency despite severely deficient (<20%) levels.
- Severe Factor XI typically causes a prolonged aPTT, but a normal aPTT may not detect a partial deficiency (FXI activity 20-60%). Evaluation should include a comprehensive bleeding history, PT/INR, and aPTT. A mixing study should be performed If aPTT is prolonged.FXI activity should be measured if FXI deficiency is suspected.
- Therapeutic challenges in managing patients with FXI deficiency include unpredictable bleeding that correlates poorly with FXI activity levels, lack of availability of FXI concentrate in many areas of the world, large volume of FFP required to achieve a hemostatic FXI activity level, and thrombotic risk associated with replacement therapy products.
- Patients with XI deficiency should ideally be managed at a hemophilia treatment center. If this is not possible, they should be managed by a hematologist experienced in managing rare bleeding disorders. Multidisciplinary care is essential to ensure optimal patient outcomes.

INTRODUCTION

Factor XI (FXI) deficiency (hemophilia C or Rosenthal disease) was first described in the 1950s by Rosenthal and colleagues[1] in four generations of a family experiencing bleeding related to surgery and dental procedures. Plasma from these patients showed correction of the clotting defect when mixed with plasma of patients with hemophilia A or B, suggesting a different factor deficiency. FXI deficiency is distinguished from FVIII deficiency (hemophilia A) and FIX deficiency (hemophilia B) by its autosomal, as opposed to X-linked, inheritance pattern and variable bleeding tendency despite severely deficient levels.

The prevalence of severe FXI deficiency is estimated to be approximately 1 in 1 million; however, it is more prevalent in the Ashkenazi and Iraqi Jewish population,

[a] Indiana Hemophilia and Thrombosis Center, 8326 Naab Road, Indianapolis, IN 46260, USA;
[b] Hematology Division, Brigham and Women's Hospital, Dana-Farber Cancer Institute, Harvard Medical School, 75 Francis Street, Boston, MA 02215, USA
* Corresponding author.
E-mail address: mlewandowska@ihtc.org
Twitter: @mlewandowskaMD (M.D.L.); @connors_md (J.M.C.)

Hematol Oncol Clin N Am 35 (2021) 1157–1169
https://doi.org/10.1016/j.hoc.2021.07.012   **hemonc.theclinics.com**
0889-8588/21/© 2021 The Authors. Published by Elsevier Inc. This is an open access article under the CC BY-NC-ND license (http://creativecommons.org/licenses/by-nc-nd/4.0/).

where heterozygosity approaches 1 in 11 (8%–9%) individuals and homozygosity/compound heterozygosity may be seen in 1 in 450 (0.2%) individuals.[2–5] Two genetic variants account for more than 90% of abnormal alleles in the Jewish population: Glu117Stop (type II) and Phe283Leu (type III).

Severe FXI deficiency is defined as activity level less than 20%, which is most commonly found in homozygotes or compound heterozygotes. Heterozygotes typically have FXI activity levels of 20% to 60%.[2,6]

The FXI gene is located on chromosome 4, and is 23 kb long. Most cases of severe deficiency seem to follow an autosomal-recessive inheritance pattern; however, a dominant-negative effect has been observed in certain heterozygous genetic variants, where a mutant FXI subunit binds to the wild-type FXI subunit, resulting in a heterodimer that cannot be secreted from the cell. This leads to lower than expected FXI activity levels.[7]

The structure of FXI has been described as a homodimeric protein comprised of two identical subunits connected by a disulfide bond (**Fig. 1**). Each subunit is comprised of four apple domains and a catalytic domain. FXI is primarily synthesized in the liver, with small quantities of transcript identified in platelets and other cell types, including islets of Langerhans in the pancreas and in renal tubule cells.[8,12]

FXI is a part of the intrinsic pathway of coagulation. It is involved in thrombin generation and the proinflammatory kallikrein-kinin system (**Fig. 2**). FXI circulates as a zymogen, and becomes activated to its enzymatic form by FXIIa, thrombin, or through autoactivation by FXIa in the presence of polyanions.

The kallikrein-kinin system consists of zymogens prekallikrein and FXII, and the cofactor high-molecular-weight kininogen. FXIIa converts FXI to FXIa. More recent coagulation models have shown that FXI is also activated by thrombin, a process that seems to be enhanced by anionic polymers, such as dextran sulfate and heparin, which are released from platelet-dense granules on activation. Prekallikrein and FXII deficiency result in prolongation in the activated partial thromboplastin time (aPTT) without associated clinical bleeding manifestations, which may be explained by the fact that FXI is also activated by thrombin.[16,17]

On activation to its enzymatic form, FXIa amplifies thrombin generation and reduces fibrinolysis. It activates FIX to FIXa, a reaction that is also catalyzed by the phospholipid-dependent FVIIa/tissue factor pathway. This dual activation of FIX to FIXa may help explain why FXI does not seem to play an integral role in thrombin generation. FXIa also activates FXII and cleaves high-molecular-weight kininogen to release bradykinin and is suspected to play a significant role in inflammatory response to injury or infection.[8,16]

CLINICAL PRESENTATION AND DIAGNOSTIC EVALUATION

Patients with FXI deficiency have an elevated aPTT; however, the bleeding tendency in FXI deficiency is generally mild, even in severe deficiency. Clinical symptoms include bleeding provoked by a surgical hemostatic challenge, postinjury, epistaxis, and heavy menstrual bleeding. Surgery involving areas with high fibrinolytic activity, such as the urogenital tract or the oropharyngeal cavity (tonsillectomy/dental extraction), seem to correlate with highest bleeding risk (49%–67%).[7] Unprovoked bleeding episodes that are frequently seen in FVIII or FIX severe deficiency, such as hemarthroses, muscle bleeds, or soft tissue bleeds, are not frequently observed in severe FXI deficiency.

Importantly, the bleeding phenotype does not correlate with the FXI activity level, with evidence of bleeding reported in heterozygotes with mild deficiency (FXI levels

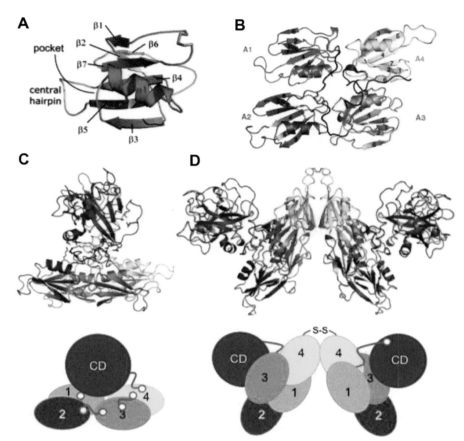

Fig. 1. (*A*) Ribbon diagram of the isolated FXI apple 1 domain from the crystal structure of the full length FXI zymogen (pdb:2F83). The α-helix is indicated in *red* and the β-sheet in *blue*. Disulfide bonds are in *yellow*. (*B*) Topology diagrams for the first, second, third, and fourth apple domains (A1, A2, A3, and A4) are shown in *gray, blue, orange,* and *yellow,* respectively. (*C*) Ribbon diagram and schematic of the FXI monomer with the catalytic domain (CD) colored *maroon* and the activation loop cleavage site residues Arg^{369}-Val^{370} colored *green*. Apple domains (numbered 1–4) are indicated by the colors described in *B*. (*D*) Ribbon diagram and schematic of the FXI dimer with the A4 domains of each subunit forming the dimer interface. The Cys^{321}-Cys^{321} bond at the top of the diagram covalently connects the subunits. (*From* Mohammed BM, Matafonov A, Ivanov I, et al. An update on factor XI structure and function. Thrombosis Research 2018;161:94-105, Emsley J, McEwan PA, Gailani D. Structure and function of factor XI. Blood 2010;115:2570, and Papagrigoriou E, McEwan PA, Walsh PN, Emsley J. Crystal structure of the factor XI zymogen reveals a pathway for transactivation. Nat Struct Mol Biol 2006;13:p.557, with permission. Mohammed et al, Emsley et al, and Papagrigoriou et al.[8–11])

20%–60%). This lack of correlation between bleeding risk and FXI activity levels poses a significant therapeutic challenge.

A study involving plasma clot structure and stability assays found that plasma from FXI-deficient patients with a clinical history of bleeding had a lower fibrin network density and lower clot stability in the presence of tissue plasminogen activator compared

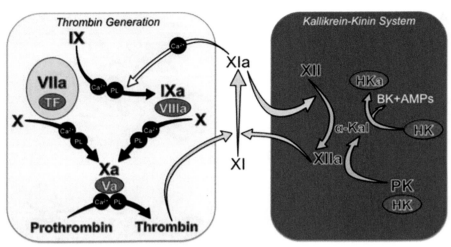

Fig. 2. *Black Roman numerals* indicate inactive zymogens of plasma proteases, and a lower-case "a" indicates active protease. Cofactors are indicated in *blue ovals*. Requirements for calcium ions (Ca2+) and phospholipid (PL) in some reactions are indicated. (*Left*) Tissue factor (TF)-initiated thrombin generation. Thrombin generation is initiated by activation of FX by the FVIIa/TF complex. FXa then converts prothrombin to thrombin in the presence of FVa. FVIIa/TF also activates FIX, and FIXa is responsible for sustaining FX and prothrombin activation.[13] The reactions indicated by the *black arrows* form the core of the thrombin generation mechanism in vertebrate animals.[14] Complete absence of one of the proteins highlighted in *red* causes either a severe bleeding disorder or is not compatible with life. FXI is a coagulation protein found only in mammals.[15] FXI provides another mechanism for FIX activation (*white arrow*) that supplements FIX activation by FVIIa/TF. It is thought that FXI is activated during hemostasis by thrombin in a reaction requiring an anionic cofactor. Polyphosphate (polymerized inorganic phosphate), which is released from platelets on activation, is a leading candidate for such a cofactor. Note that FXI during hemostasis is not thought to require FXIIa. (*Right*) Contact activation (kallikrein-kinin system). Exposure of blood to a variety of artificial and biologic surfaces triggers contact activation. FXII and prekallikrein (PK) bind to the surface and convert each other to FXIIa and α-kallikrein. High-molecular-weight kininogen (HK) is a cofactor for the reaction, facilitating PK binding to the surface. FXIIa can activate FXI leading to thrombin generation. There is also evidence that FXIa, like α-kallikrein, can activate FXII. Contact activation triggers thrombin generation in the activated partial thromboplastin time assay, but it is doubtful that it contributes to hemostasis, because congenital FXII, PK, or HK deficiency does not cause a bleeding disorder. Because of this, FXII, PK, and HK are often considered to form a system separate from FXI referred to as the kallikrein-kinin system (KKS components highlighted in *yellow*). Activation of the KKS results in cleavage of HK by α-kallikrein generating the potent vasoactive peptide bradykinin (BK) and antimicrobial peptides (AMPs) that likely play a role in host defense. In this figure, *gray arrows* indicate reactions that are enhanced by polyanions, such as polyphosphate, DNA, and RNA. (*From* Wheeler AP, Gailani D. Why factor XI deficiency is a clinical concern. Expert Rev Hematol 2016;9:629-37; with permission.)

with their FXI-deficient counterparts without a history of bleeding.[18] A recent study also found that the degree to which individuals are able to generate thrombin in platelet-rich plasma with low tissue factor concentration and inhibition of contact activation differentiated bleeding phenotype.[19] Furthermore, the effectiveness of tranexamic acid and ε-aminocaproic acid in treatment of bleeding episodes in FXI-deficient patients suggests that FXI plays a significant role in preventing premature fibrinolysis.

Diagnostic evaluation should include a comprehensive bleeding history and laboratory evaluation, including prothrombin time (PT) and aPTT. If the PT or aPTT are prolonged, a mixing study is performed. Correction to the normal range is consistent with a factor deficiency. FXI deficiency typically causes a prolonged aPTT in the setting of a normal PT, FVIII activity, and FIX activity. In general, the aPTT is prolonged when the FXI activity level is decreased less than 30%.[9] Different aPTT reagents may have variable sensitivity to FXI deficiency. Whereas a normal aPTT excludes severe FXI deficiency, it may not detect a partial deficiency (FXI activity 20%–60%), which may still be associated with clinical bleeding complications. Evaluation of the coagulation factors in the intrinsic pathway despite a normal aPTT is encouraged in the appropriate clinical setting, and FXI-specific activity should be measured if FXI deficiency is suspected.

MANAGEMENT

Therapeutic agents available for management of FXI deficiency include fresh frozen plasma (FFP), FXI concentrates (currently available in certain European countries), and low-dose recombinant factor VIIa (rVIIa). Antifibrinolytic agents, such as ε-aminocaproic acid or tranexamic acid, may be used for treatment of minor bleeding episodes or perioperatively for certain surgeries. Antibrinolytic agents may also be used as adjunctive therapy to other hemostatic agents.

FXI has a half-life of approximately 50 to 70 hours.[20–22] As such, exogenous FXI replacement with FFP or FXI concentrate may be administered every 48 to 72 hours. Several studies have demonstrated the safety and efficacy of low-dose rFVIIa for perioperative management of patients with FXI deficiency. Use of these lower doses of rFVIIa (15–20 μg/kg) may reduce thrombotic risk.[5,23]

Patients with FXI deficiency should receive genetic counseling and education on bleeding risks and inhibitor development. Genetic testing should be offered to affected individuals and first-degree relatives. Antithrombotic agents, such as anticoagulants and antiplatelet medications, should generally be avoided; if these agents are required for treatment of another medical condition, consultation with a hemophilia treatment center or hematologists with experience managing FXI is advised.

Clinical challenges that remain in the management of patients with FXI deficiency include unpredictable bleeding that does not correlate well with FXI activity level, the large volume of FFP required to achieve a hemostatic level, lack of availability of an FXI concentrate that is safe and effective in all regions, and thrombotic risk with existing replacement therapy products (**Table 1**).

SPECIAL POPULATIONS
Homozygotes for Factor XI Deficiency

In general, the severity of FXI deficiency does not correlate well with clinical bleeding manifestations[30]; however, certain FXI mutations seem to have somewhat higher phenotypic correlation. Severe FXI deficiency is defined as an activity level less than 20%; however, certain genetic variants confer a lower FXI activity level. Many homozygous-deficient patients have FXI activity levels less than 1%.

The Glu117Stop (type II) mutation introduces a premature termination codon in the apple 2 domain, with homozygotes exhibiting FXI activity levels of less than 1%. Patients with FXI activity of less than 1% are at significant risk for developing neutralizing antibodies. The Phe283Leu (type III) mutation occurs in the apple 4 domain, which interferes with dimer formation and reduces protein secretion; typically homozygotes have baseline FXI activity levels of about 10%.[31,32]

Table 1
Products available for treatment of FXI deficiency[5,16]

Product	Dose (Adult)	Indications	Adverse Reactions
FFP (SD treated)[5,22]	15–20 mL/kg[22]	Major hemostatic challenge (ie, surgery) in appropriate clinical setting	Volume overload Hypersensitivity reaction Risk of inhibitor development
aFXI concentrate[5,22]	15–20 U/kg increase FXI activity by ~30% Dose of FXI (units) = weight (kg) × (goal FXI level - baseline FXI level) × 0.5. Repeat every 48–72 h as needed	Major hemostatic challenge (ie, surgery) in appropriate clinical setting	Risk of inhibitor development Thrombotic risk[24]
rFVIIa[5,23]	15–20 µg/kg in conjunction with TXA	Major hemostatic challenge in the setting of FXI deficiency and/or active inhibitor High inhibitor risk (ie, homozygous Glu117Stop), desire to avoid exogenous FXI exposure	Thrombotic risk at higher doses (90 µg/kg) Note: Not FDA approved for treatment of FXI deficiency
Tranexamic acid[25–27]	PO: 1300 mg 3 times daily (adult) 15–20 mg/kg every 8 h (pediatric) IV: 10 mg/kg every 6–8 h	Prevention of postpartum bleeding Heavy menstrual bleeding (~5–7 d) Oral cavity bleeding Adjunctive treatment with FFP/FXI concentrate/rFVIIa for major hemostatic challenge	Thrombosis Avoid in GU tract bleeding
ε-Aminocaproic acid[28,29]	PO: Adult: 3 g 4 times daily Pediatric: 100 mg/kg PO every 6 h IV: Adult: 4–5 g during first h, followed by 1 g/h × 8 h	Prevention of postpartum bleeding Heavy menstrual bleeding Oral cavity bleeding Adjunctive treatment with FFP/FXI concentrate/rFVIIa for major hemostatic challenge	Thrombosis Avoid in GU tract bleeding

Abbreviations: EACA, Epsilon aminocaproic acid; FDA, Food and Drug Administration; FFP, fresh frozen plasma; GU, genitourinary; IV, intravenous; SD, solvent detergent TXA, tranexamic acid.

a Most experts suggest trough FXI activity level of approximately 30 to 45 should be sufficient for hemostasis in patients with severe activity. Plasma FXI activity should not exceed 70 IU/dL, because this may increase thrombotic risk.[6]

Data from Ponchek M, Shamanaev A, et al. The evolution of FXI and the kallikrein-kinin system. *Blood Advances.* 2020 Dec; 4 (24): 6135-6147 and Bolton-Maggs PH, Shapiro AD, et al. Rare Coagulation Disorders Resource Room. Available at: https://www.rarecoagulationdisorders.org/. Accessed February 23, 2021.

Inhibitors

FXI inhibitors are alloantibodies that develop in response to exogenous FXI exposure, which may occur in approximately 10% of severely FXI-deficient patients. Specific genotypes are associated with an increased risk of inhibitor development. Individuals homozygous for the Glu117Stop (type II) genetic variant have an up to 30% risk of inhibitor development in some reports.[31] In these individuals, the use of FFP and FXI concentrates should be judicious. FXI inhibitors have not been described in partial deficiency (FXI activity >20%).

Spontaneous bleeding is rare despite the presence of FXI inhibitors, and may only manifest with severe bleeding after a significant hemostatic challenge, such as surgery or trauma. Close monitoring for FXI inhibitors is prudent after exogenous FXI replacement, especially in homozygotes for the type II genetic variant. For patients requiring therapy, the preferred treatment is low-dose rFVIIa and antifibrinolytic therapy.[23,33–36] Treatment to eradicate inhibitors to FXI is usually clinically unnecessary, as patients generally do not develop spontaneous bleeding symptoms.

WOMEN'S HEALTH
Case 1

A 30-year-old G1P0 woman is 35 weeks pregnant. She is referred for evaluation of a possible bleeding disorder in anticipation of upcoming delivery with planned neuraxial anesthesia. Her past medical history includes heavy menstrual bleeding with resultant iron deficiency anemia and epistaxis requiring nasal cautery. Laboratory evaluation reveals a prolonged aPTT at 63 seconds that corrects to 25 seconds on mixing study. FVIII activity, FIX activity, and Von Willebrand disease studies are normal. FXI activity is 11 IU/dL. What is the best recommendation for management around the time of delivery?

Answer

Given the severity of the patient's FXI deficiency and personal bleeding history, FXI-replacement therapy with either FFP or FXI concentrate is indicated before administration of neuraxial anesthesia. Postpartum antifibrinolytic therapy should also be considered.

Heavy menstrual bleeding is frequent in women with FXI deficiency. In a study reported by Kadir and colleagues,[37] 59% of women with FXI deficiency endorsed heavy menstrual bleeding, compared with 10% of the general population. Treatment options for heavy menstrual bleeding include antifibrinolytic therapy (tranexamic acid, ε-aminocaproic acid) and hormonal-suppressive therapy.

Postpartum hemorrhage (PPH) has been reported in women with mild and severe FXI deficiency, leading to a debate regarding the need for replacement therapy before delivery. For women with levels less than 1%, replacement using FFP or FXI concentrate is appropriate in preparation for delivery. If using FFP, 20 mL/kg may be needed to achieve a level of approximately 25%, which normalizes the aPTT.

A recent retrospective, case-control study in women with FXI levels between 20% and 70% found no cases of PPH among 45 vaginal deliveries, which was not statistically different compared with the control group without FXI deficiency (1/125). Only 1 patient with FXI deficiency received treatment with FFP prior to delivery. Conversely, 38% (10/26) of women with FXI deficiency undergoing caesarian section developed PPH, compared with 18.7% (14/75) of the control group (odds ratio, 2.73; 95% confidence interval, 1.02–7.26; $P = .04$).[38] Seventy percent of women who developed PPH had a prior personal history of bleeding; in contrast, FXI levels did not seem predictive of PPH.

In the same study,[38] neuraxial anesthesia was used in 51 patients with mild FXI deficiency, with no observed complications. Only three patients received prophylaxis with FFP, one of whom also received antifibrinolytic therapy. Another case series authored by Singh and colleagues[39] described experience managing 13 FXI-deficient patients around delivery; nine patients received neuraxial anesthesia without complication (epidural, seven; spinal, one; combined spinal-epidural, one). Five of these patients were treated with FFP before anesthetic administration; the ones who did not receive FFP had mild FXI deficiency and no personal history of bleeding.

A detailed assessment of personal bleeding history (ie, ISTH-BAT)[40] and family history of bleeding therefore may be helpful in determining the need for factor replacement therapy before delivery. The use of antifibrinolytic therapy should be considered in the postpartum setting.

Neonatal bleeding is rare, but instrumentation (ie, vacuum, forceps delivery) should generally be avoided in all known affected or potentially affected infants. Cord blood measurement of FXI activity should be performed, particularly in males for whom circumcision is being considered.

A multidisciplinary approach should be used, involving hematology, obstetrics/gynecology, and anesthesia in preparation for delivery to optimize patient care.

PERIOPERATIVE MANAGEMENT
Case 2

A 35-year-old man with known severe (<1 IU/dL) FXI deficiency presents for evaluation before an upcoming dental extraction. Genetic testing reveals homozygosity for the Glu117Stop (type II) variant. What treatment would you recommend periprocedurally?

Answer

Individuals homozygous for the Glu117Stop (type II) genetic variant have an up to 30% risk of inhibitor development, therefore exposure to FXI should be avoided whenever possible. Given that a dental extraction is a minor hemostatic challenge, it is reasonable to plan for single-agent antifibrinolytic therapy with either tranexamic acid or ε-aminocaproic acid for 5 to 7 days following dental extraction; in the event of unexpected or breakthrough bleeding, low-dose rFVIIa may be used.

Investigators have reported postoperative bleeding in greater than 60% of severe FXI-deficient patients who underwent oropharyngeal or urologic surgery.[31]

Patients with FXI activity level of less than 20% who are undergoing major surgery should receive FXI-replacement therapy, with a goal FXI trough activity level 30% to 45%. Major surgery in areas of increased fibrinolytic activity may require higher trough levels of 45 IU/DL for 5 to 7 days.[6] Plasma FXI activity should not exceed 70 IU/dL, because this may increase thrombotic risk. Whenever possible, perioperative management should include close collaboration with a hemophilia treatment center. The ability to perform routine measurement of FXI activity levels is imperative to ensure proper dosing for therapeutic levels.

A detailed individual bleeding history is essential. A lack of bleeding with prior hemostatic challenges does not always exclude the risk of hemorrhage with future surgical procedures. In individuals who are homozygous for the Glu117Stop variant, FXI replacement should be reserved for major hemostatic challenges due to increased risk of inhibitor development.

Cardiovascular evaluation is indicated in patients for whom the use of FFP is being considered, because of the potential for volume overload. For severely deficient patients, it may take 1000 to 1500 mL of FFP to achieve an acceptable level of FXI to achieve hemostasis for major surgery. Thrombotic risk factors should be considered in patients for whom treatment with FXI concentrate or rFVIIa is being considered; these include personal risk factors for thrombosis, surgical thrombotic risk, and family history of thrombosis. There are two FXI concentrates, FXI BPL and Hemoleven LFB, neither of which is currently available in the United States.

Recombinant FVIIa (rFVIIa) has been used perioperatively in patients with congenital FXI deficiency and an inhibitor. An increased thrombotic risk has been reported when doses of rFVIIa of approximately 90 µg/kg were administered.[36] Several subsequent studies in FXI-deficient patients with inhibitors documented that using a single infusion of low-dose rFVIIa (15–30 µg/kg) with adjunctive tranexamic acid (TXA) starting 2 hours before surgery and continued until 7 to 14 days postoperatively seemed to provide adequate hemostasis without excessive bleeding or thrombotic episodes.[23,33] Given the short half-life of rFVIIa (~4–6 hours), repeat administration may be necessary depending on clinical bleeding manifestations. In addition, the successful use of low-dose rFVIIa in FXI-deficient patients without inhibitors who desired to avoid plasma products has also been reported, without reported thrombotic complications.[35] This may be a reasonable approach to consider in patients with high risk of inhibitor development (ie, homozygous Glu117Stop genetic variant). rFVIIa is not Food and Drug Administration approved for treatment or prevention of bleeding in the setting of FXI deficiency.

Antifibrinolytic agents (tranexamic acid, ε-aminocaproic acid) may be a useful adjunctive treatment for surgical procedures. Treatment with single-agent antifibrinolytic therapy may also be effective in minor procedures involving fibrin-rich tissue, such as dental extractions or other procedures involving mucosal tissue.

TARGETING FACTOR XI AS AN ANTICOAGULANT

Widespread use of direct oral anticoagulants has ushered in a new era of anticoagulation. Despite improvement in bleeding risk compared with vitamin K antagonist therapy, excessive bleeding risk remains a clinical concern. FXII and FXI are attractive targets, because they seem to be integral in thrombus stabilization, but do not seem to be vital for hemostasis. Spontaneous bleeding in FXI deficiency is rare. In animal models, FXI or FXII deficiency seems to confer protection against thrombosis. Mice with FXI or FXII deficiency had decreased risk of ischemic stroke and thrombosis after venous flow restriction, and FXI or FXII knockdown rabbits with antisense oligonucleotides (ASOs) had a reduced rate of catheter thrombosis.[41–43]

Several strategies for targeting FXI have been developed. ASOs reduce hepatic synthesis of FXI by inducing degradation of FXI mRNA.[43–45] Monoclonal antibodies block FXI activation or inhibit FXIa activity.[46] Aptamers bind FXI or FXIa.[45,47] Small peptidomimetic molecules reversibly bind to the catalytic domain of FXIa, thereby inhibiting its activity.[48–51]

Monoclonal antibodies, aptamers, and small molecules have a rapid onset of action, whereas the onset of action of ASOs is prolonged at 3 to 4 weeks. Small peptidomimetic molecules also have the potential for oral administration, whereas ASOs, antibodies, and aptamers are administered parenterally.

ASO therapy aimed at reducing FXI levels was evaluated in a phase 2 trial to prevent venous thrombosis after knee replacement; no excessive bleeding was reported.[52] A total of 300 patients were randomized to receive enoxaparin postoperative or IONIS-416858 (either 200 mg or 300 mg) beginning 35 days before surgery. Treatment was continued for at least 10 days postoperatively. The primary outcome of venous thromboembolism occurred in 36/134 patients (27%) patients receiving 200 mg of IONIS-

416858, 3/71 (4%) patients receiving 300 mg of IONIS-416858, and 21/69 (30%) patients who received enoxaparin. There was no statistically significant difference in bleeding (3% in both IONIS-416858 groups, 8% in the enoxaparin group). Additionally, there are two studies ongoing to evaluate the safety of IONIS-416858 in patients on hemodialysis to evaluate reduction of dialysis circuit clotting events (URL: https://www.clinicaltrials.gov. Unique identifiers: NCT02553889 and NCT03358030).

The recently published phase 2 FOXTROT trial evaluated the use of a fully human monoclonal immunoglobulin G1 antibody targeting FXI, osocimab, in preventing venous thromboembolism among patients undergoing knee arthroplasty. Osocimab has a half-life of 30-44 days and is given as an intravenous infusion. The primary outcome was the incidence of venous thromboembolism at 10 to 13 days postoperatively. A total of 814 patients were randomized to receive postoperative enoxaparin, postoperative apixaban, postoperative osocimab (0.3 mg/kg, 0.6 mg/kg, 1.2 mg/kg, or 1.8 mg/kg), or preoperative osocimab (0.3 mg/kg or 1.8 mg/kg). Enoxaparin 40 mg was given subcutaneously once daily starting the evening before surgery or 6 to 8 hours postoperatively (at the investigator's discretion). Apixaban 2.5 mg twice daily was given orally twice daily beginning 12 to 24 hours postoperatively. Enoxaparin and apixaban were continued for at least 10 days or until venography was performed 10 to 13 days postoperatively. The postoperative osocimab groups receiving 0.6 mg/kg, 1.2 mg/kg, and 1.8 mg/kg met criteria for noninferiority; the preoperative 1.8 mg/kg dose of osocimab met criteria for superiority. The 0.3 mg/kg osocimab preoperative or postoperative groups did not meet criteria for noninferiority compared with postoperative enoxaparin or apixaban. Overall, osocimab seemed safe and effective compared with prophylactic dose enoxaparin and apixaban.[15]

Another phase II study is evaluating BMS986177, an oral FXIa inhibitor, for prevention of new ischemic stroke or new covert brain infarction in patients receiving aspirin and clopidogrel following acute ischemic stroke or transient ischemic attack (URL: https://www.clinicaltrials.gov. Unique identifier: NCT03766581).

SUMMARY

FXI deficiency is a rare autosomal coagulation factor deficiency that is usually associated with bleeding only in the setting of invasive procedures and trauma, although in women it can manifest as heavy menstrual bleeding. Personal and family history of bleeding should be ascertained and can help guide perioperative management and the need for FXI replacement therapy. Coordination of care between hematologists, anesthesiologists, and obstetricians or surgeons is crucial to ensure optimal patient care. The lack of spontaneous bleeding associated with FXI deficiency has made this coagulation factor an attractive target to inhibit to prevent thrombosis while preserving hemostasis. Results from trials that are underway should be forthcoming in the next few years.

CLINICS CARE POINTS

- FXI deficiency (Hemophilia C or Rosenthal's disease) is predominantly an autosomal-recessive trait, although some mutations follow an autosomal-dominant inheritance pattern.
- Patients with FIX deficiency demonstrate variable bleeding tendency despite severe deficiency (FXI activity <20%).
- Clinical symptoms include bleeding provoked by a surgical hemostatic challenge, post-injury, epistaxis, and heavy menstrual bleeding. Surgery involving highly fibrinolytic (ie. urogenital, oropharyngeal) areas confers a higher bleeding risk.

- Individuals homozygous for the Glu117Stop (Type II) genetic variant have an up to 30% risk of inhibitor development, therefore exposure to FXI should be avoided whenever possible.

- A detailed personal and family history of bleeding may be helpful in determining the need for factor replacement therapy prior to surgery or delivery.

- Treatment options include FXI concentrate (not currently available in the U.S.), FFP, and adjunctive antifibrinolytics. Low dose rFVIIa may be used in patients with inhibitors to FXI and may be considered in patients with high inhibitor risk who wish to avoid exposure to exogenous FXI.

DISCLOSURE

M.D. Lewandowska: Advisory board for Bio Products Laboratory. All Honoraria donated to the Indiana Hemophilia and Thrombosis Center. J.M. Connors: No relationships to disclose related to this article; others include personal fees for scientific Ad Boards and Consulting: Abbott, Anthos, Alnylam, Bristol-Myers Squibb, Portola, and Takeda. Research funding to the institution from CSL Behring.

REFERENCES

1. Rosenthal RL, Dreskin OH, et al. New hemophilia-like disease caused by deficiency of a third plasma thromboplastin factor. Proc Soc Exp Biol Med 1953; 82:171–4.
2. Shapiro AD, Heiman M, et al. Gene test interpretation: F11 (gene for coagulation factor XI). UpToDate. Leung LLK, editor. Waltham (MA) 2021. Available at: https://www.uptodate.com/contents/gene-test-interpretation-f11-gene-for-coagulation-factor-xi?search=FGene%20test%20interpretation:%20F11%20Shapiro&source=search_result&selectedTitle=1~150&usage_type=default&display_rank=1. Accessed February 23, 2021.
3. Gerber GF, Klute KA, et al. Peri- and postpartum management of patients with factor XI deficiency. Clin Appl Thromb Hemost 2019;25:1–8.
4. Duga S, Salomon O. Congenital factor XI deficiency: an update. Semin Thromb Hemost 2013;39(6):621–31.
5. Bolton-Maggs PH, Shapiro AD, et al. Rare coagulation disorders resource room. Available at: https://www.rarecoagulationdisorders.org/. Accessed February 23, 2021.
6. Bolton-Maggs PHB. Factor XI deficiency—resolving the enigma? Hematology 2009;2009(1):97–105.
7. Kravtsov DV, Wu W, Meijers JC, et al. Dominant factor XI deficiency caused by mutations in the factor XI catalytic domain. Blood 2004;104(1):128–34.
8. Mohammed BM, Matanfonov A, et al. Thromb Res 2018;161:94–105.
9. Papagrigoriou E, McEwan PA, Walsh PN, et al. Crystal structure of the factor XI zymogen reveals a pathway for transactivation. Nat Struct Mol Biol 2006;13(6):557–8.
10. Emsley J, McEwan PA, Gailani D. Structure and function of factor XI. Blood 2010; 115(13):2569–77.
11. Asakai R, Davie EW, et al. Organization of the gene for human factor XI. Biochemistry 1987;26:7221–8.
12. Buller HR, Bethune C, et al. Factor XI antisense oligonucleotide for prevention of venous thrombosis. N Engl J Med 2015;373(3):232–40.
13. Salomon O, Zivelin A, et al. Prevalence, causes, and characterization of factor XI inhibitors in patients with inherited factor XI deficiency. Blood 2003;101(12):4783.

14. Kagdi H, Ling G, et al. Safety and efficacy of factor XI (FXI) concentrate use in patients with FXI deficiency: a single-centre experience of 19 years. Haemophilia 2015;22(3):411–8.

15. Weitz JI, Bauersachs R. Effect of osocimab in preventing venous thromboembolism among patients undergoing knee arthroplasty, the FOXTROT randomized clinical trial. JAMA 2020;323(2):130–9.

16. Ponchek M, Shamanaev A, et al. The evolution of factor XI and the kallikrein-kinin system. Blood Adv 2020;4(24):6135–47.

17. Wheeler AP, Gailani D. Why factor XI deficiency is a clinical concern. Expert Rev Hematol 2016;9(7):629–37.

18. Zucker M, Seligsohn U, et al. Abnormal plasma clot structure and stability distinguish bleeding risk in patients with severe factor XI deficiency. J Thromb Haemost 2014;12(7):1121–30.

19. Gidley GN, Holle LA, et al. Abnormal plasma clot formation and fibrinolysis reveal bleeding tendency in patients with partial factor XI deficiency. Blood Adv 2018;2: 1076–88.

20. Nossel HL, Niemetz J, et al. Blood PTA (factor XI) levels following plasma infusion. Pro Soc Exp Biol Med 1964;115:896–897n.

21. Palla R, Peyvandi F, et al. Rare bleeding disorders: diagnosis and treatment. Blood 2015;125(13):2052–61.

22. Peyvandi F, Palla R, et al. European Network of Rare Bleeding Disorders group coagulation factor activity and clinical bleeding severity in rare bleeding disorders: results from the European Network of Rare Bleeding Disorders. J Thromb Haemost 2012;10(4):615–21.

23. Livnat T, Tamarin I, et al. Recombinant activated factor VII and tranexamic acid are haemostatically effective during major surgery in factor XI-deficient patients with inhibitor antibodies. Thromb Haemost 2009;102(3):487.

24. Bolton-Maggs PH, Goudemand J, et al. FXI concentrate and risk of thrombosis. Haemophilia 2014;20(4):e349–51.

25. Cyklokapron (tranexamic acid) (prescribing information). New York: Pharmacia & Upjohn Company; 2021.

26. WOMAN trial collaborators. Effect of early tranexamic acid administration on mortality, hysterectomy, and other morbidities in women with post-partum haemorrhage (WOMAN): an international, randomised, double-blind, placebo-controlled trial. Lancet 2017;389(10084):2105–16 [published correction appears in Lancet. 2017;389(10084):2104].

27. Lysteda (tranexamic acid) (prescribing information). Parsippany (NJ): Ferring Pharmaceuticals Inc; 2020.

28. Amicar (aminocaproic acid) [prescribing information]. Lake Forest (IL): Clover Pharmaceuticals; 2017.

29. Aminocaproic acid injection solution [prescribing information]. Lehi (UT): Civica, Inc; 2020.

30. Bolton-Maggs PH, Patterson DA, et al. Definition of the bleeding tendency in factor XI-deficient kindreds: a clinical and laboratory study. Thromb Haemost 1995; 73:194–202.

31. Asakai R, Chung DW, et al. Factor XI deficiency in Ashkenazi Jews in Israel. N Engl J Med 1991;325:153–8.

32. Salomon O, Steinberg DM, et al. Variable bleeding manifestations characterize different types of surgery in patients with severe factor XI deficiency enabling parsimonious use of replacement therapy. Hemophilia 2006;12:490–3.

33. Salomon O, Tamarin I, et al. Patients with severe factor XI deficiency who have an inhibitor or IgA deficiency can undergo uneventful major surgery by a single infusion of low dose recombinant factor VIIa and use of tranexamic acid. Blood 2008; 112(11):1215.
34. O'Connell NM, Riddell AF, et al. Recombinant factor VIIa to prevent surgical bleeding in factor XI deficiency. Haemophilia 2008;14:775–81.
35. Riddell A, Abdul-Kadir R, et al. Monitoring low dose recombinant factor VIIa therapy in patients with severe factor XI deficiency undergoing surgery. J Thromb Haemost 2011;106(3):521–7.
36. O'Connell NM. Factor XI deficiency. Semin Hematol 2004;41(1 Suppl 1):76.
37. Kadir RA, Economides DL, et al. Factor XI deficiency in women. Am J Hematol 1999;60:48–54.
38. Stoeckle JH, Bogue T, et al. Postpartum haemorrhage in women with mild factor XI deficiency. Haemophilia 2020;26(4):663–6.
39. Singh A, Harnett M, Connors J, et al. Factor XI deficiency and obstetrical anesthesia. Anesth Analg 2009;108(6):1882–5.
40. Rodeghiero F, Tosetto A, et al. ISTH/SSC bleeding assessment tool: a standardized questionnaire and a proposal for a new bleeding score for inherited bleeding disorders. ISTH/SSC joint VWF and Perinatal/Pediatric Hemostasis Subcommittees Working Group. J Thromb Haemost 2010;8(9):2063–5.
41. Renné T, Oschatz C, et al. Factor XI deficiency in animal models. J Thromb Haemost 2009;7(Suppl 1):79–83.
42. Revenko AS, Gao D, et al. Selective depletion of plasma prekallikrein or coagulation factor XII inhibits thrombosis in mice without increased risk of bleeding. Blood 2011;118:5302–11.
43. Yau JW, Liao P, et al. Selective depletion of factor XI or factor XII with antisense oligonucleotides attenuates catheter thrombosis in rabbits. Blood 2014;123:2102–7.
44. Zhang H, Löwenberg EC, et al. Inhibition of the intrinsic coagulation pathway factor XI by antisense oligonucleotides: a novel antithrombotic strategy with lowered bleeding risk. Blood 2010;116:4684–92.
45. Weitz JI, Chan NC. Advances in antithrombotic therapy. Arterioscler Thromb Vasc Biol 2019;39:7–12.
46. Tucker EI, Marzec UM, et al. Prevention of vascular graft occlusion and thrombus-associated thrombin generation by inhibition of factor XI. Blood 2009;113:936–44.
47. Woodruff RS, Ivanov, et al. Generation and characterization of aptamers targeting factor XIa. Thromb Res 2017;156:134–41.
48. Lin J, Deng H, et al. Design, synthesis, and biological evaluation of peptidomimetic inhibitors of factor XIa as novel anticoagulants. J Med Chem 2006;49:7781–91.
49. Perera V, Luettgen JM, et al. First-in-human study to assess the safety, pharmacokinetics and pharmacodynamics of BMS-962212, a direct, reversible, small molecule factor XIa inhibitor in non-Japanese and Japanese healthy subjects. Br J Clin Pharmacol 2018;84:876–87.
50. Wong PC, Crain EJ, et al. A small-molecule factor XIa inhibitor produces antithrombotic efficacy with minimal bleeding time prolongation in rabbits. J Thromb Thrombolysis 2011;32:129–37.
51. Al-Horani RA, Ponnusamy P, et al. Sulfated pentagalloylglucoside is a potent, allosteric, and selective inhibitor of factor XIa. J Med Chem 2013;56:867–78.
52. Buller HR, Bethune C, et al. Factor XI antisense oligonucleotide for prevention of venous thrombosis. N Engl J Med 2015;372:232–40.

Factor XIII Deficiency
A Review of Clinical Presentation and Management

Ari Pelcovits, MD[a,b], Fred Schiffman, MD[a,b], Rabin Niroula, MD[a,b],*

KEYWORDS

- FXIII deficiency • Rare bleeding disorder • Hemophilia

KEY POINTS

- Factor XIII deficiency can result in life-threatening bleeding and requires prophylactic management for patients with activity levels less than 5%.
- Women with factor XIII deficiency require replacement therapy during pregnancy to increase fetal vitality.
- Plasma concentrate–derived and recombinant factor XIII replacement therapies exist, although only plasma-derived therapy can be used for deficiencies of the B subunit.

INTRODUCTION

Factor XIII (FXIII) deficiency is a rare autosomal recessive disorder that can result in life-threatening bleeding and early fetal loss.[1,2] FXIII is responsible for cross-linking fibrinogen to stabilize and strengthen clot formation, facilitates wound healing and angiogenesis, and plays an important role in fetal vitality.[3]

This article reviews the history, clinical features, diagnosis, and treatment of FXIII deficiency. Its discovery, biochemical function, and classical clinical phenotype are highlighted and recent therapeutic options discussed.

BACKGROUND

FXIII first was identified in 1944 as a plasma protein that was essential for fibrin stabilization and initially was coined fibrin stabilization factor.[3] In 1968, FXIII was shown conclusively to function as a transglutaminase, forming bonds between glutamine and lysine side chains of fibrin monomers.[4] A majority of the other coagulation proteins, besides factor V and factor VIII, which are glycoproteins, are serine proteases,

a Alpert Medical School of Brown University, Providence, RI, USA; b Division of Hematology-Oncology, Rhode Island Hospital and The Miriam Hospital, 164 Summit Avenue, Providence, RI 02906, USA
* Corresponding author. Warren Alpert Medical School of Brown University, Rhode Island Hospital, 593 Eddy Street, Providence, RI 02903.
E-mail address: Rabin_Niroula@brown.edu

Hematol Oncol Clin N Am 35 (2021) 1171–1180
https://doi.org/10.1016/j.hoc.2021.07.009
0889-8588/21/© 2021 Elsevier Inc. All rights reserved.

waiting to be activated themselves before cleaving and activating the next step in the coagulation cascade. FXIII then has a unique enzymatic function in the coagulation pathway.

In plasma, FXIII circulates as a pro-transglutaminase (FXIII-AB) composed of 2 catalytic A subunits (FXIII-A) and 2 noncatalytic B subunits (FXIII-B) held together by noncovalent bonds. FXIII requires cleavage by thrombin for the formation of FXIIIa, the enzymatic portion of the protein.[3] The A subunits are synthesized by hematopoietic cells, whereas liver is the major site of B subunit synthesis. They are coded by different genes, chromosome 6 (*F13A*) and chromosome 1 (*F13B*), respectively.[3] Congenital FXIII deficiency is caused by defects in either FXIII-A subunit gene or FXIII-B subunit gene. The bleeding disorder resulting from mutations in FXIII-B occurs infrequently (<5% of reported cases of FXIII deficiency cases) and is less severe in general.[5]

EPIDEMIOLOGY AND SYMPTOMATOLOGY
Congenital Factor XIII Deficiency

Congenital FXIII deficiency is a rare genetic condition, with an incidence of 1 in approximately 2 million people worldwide. It is one of the rarest causes of inherited bleeding disorders and is part of the group of rare inherited bleeding disorders that include deficiencies in factors X, VII, V, II and XIII. FXIII deficiency accounts for approximately 6% of these cases of rare inherited bleeding disorders.[6] This rare bleeding disorder affects people of all races and ethnicities and is inherited in an autosomal recessive pattern. There often is a history of consanguinity within certain families of FXIII-deficient patients. However, non-cansanguineous inheritance is seen as well.[7]

Patients with FXIII deficiency often are diagnosed after presenting with severe bleeding and poor wound healing. Female patients sometimes are diagnosed later in life after unexplained multiple miscarriages.[8] Clinical presentation and common sites of bleeding are extrapolated from case series and patient registries, a series of which are listed in **Table 1**. Delayed umbilical cord stump bleeding is the most common presenting symptom in neonates.[1] Bleeding episodes can be life threatening and include intracranial bleeding, delayed umbilical stump bleeding, musculocutaneous bleeding, hemarthrosis, and posttraumatic or postsurgical bleeding (see **Table 1**).

FXIII deficiency also appears uniquely associated with pregnancy loss among the rare bleeding disorders. In one review of multiple case reports and case series that included 121 women with FXIII deficiency, 66% of all pregnancies resulted in a miscarriage.[2] Although the number of patients was limited, the rates of miscarriage were higher in women with a deficiency in the A subunit (70%) as opposed to the B subunit (15%; 2 of 13 pregnancies). Although the exact reason for an increased rate of miscarriages in patients with FXIII deficiency is unknown, this is consistent with preclinical work that showed a unique role of FXIII A subunit in fetal viability, specifically in preventing intrauterine bleeding.[9] Alternatively, FXIII-A also may play a role in placental adhesion and implantation.[10]

The level of FXIII activity correlates with bleeding severity. In a 2012 study using data from 489 patients registered in the European Network of Rare Bleeding Disorders, including 42 patients with FXIII deficiency, there was a strong association between bleeding severity and factor activity level.[11] Although patients with FXIII activity level of greater than or equal to 30 IU dL^{-1} (equivalent to $\geq$30% activity level) remained largely asymptomatic, and patients with undetectable levels had high rates of grade III bleeding, there was significant variability between these levels with regard to bleeding severity (see **Table 1** for bleeding grade descriptions).

Table 1
Studies of clinical bleeding manifestations of factor XIII deficiency

Year Published	2003[27]	2004[28]	2007[29]	2012[11]	2012[30]	2016[1]	2017[12]	2020[8]
Number of patients	93	33	104	42	88	317	64	33
Locations of bleeding								
Subcutaneous	58%[d]	47%[a]	57%		56%	—		—
Umbilical stump	73%	22%	56%		83%	77.3%		57.6%
Muscle	—	27%	49%		—	—		—
Postoperative	84%[c]	4%	40%		—	—		—
Trauma	—		—		77%	—		18.2%
Hemarthrosis	55%		36%		9%	—		3.2%
Intracranial	25%	10%	34%		13%	45.7%		27.3%
Mucosal	48%	47%[a]	—		32%	—		
Severity of bleeding[b]								
Asymptomatic				39.3%			9%[e]	
Grade I				6.1%			16%	
Grade II				6.1%			12%	
Grade III				48.5%			55%	

[a] Mucocutaneous listed as 1 category and did not differentiate between skin and mucous membrane bleeding.
[b] Asymptomatic: no documented bleeding; grade I: occurred after trauma or drug ingestion (antiplatelet or anticoagulant therapy); grade II: spontaneous minor bleeding: bruising, ecchymosis, minor wounds, oral cavity bleeding, epistaxis, and menorrhagia; and grade III: spontaneous major bleeding: hematomas, hemarthrosis, central nervous system, gastrointestinal, and umbilical cord stump bleeding.
[c] Of patients who underwent surgery without prophylactic treatment who required blood transfusions.
[d] Hematoma.
[e] Another 8% bled only during pregnancy.

The correlation of activity level with bleeding was confirmed in a 2017 cross-sectional study of FXIII-deficient patients identified in the Prospective Rare Bleeding Disorders Database, a worldwide database of patients with rare bleeding disorders.[12] Of 64 patients identified in this study, all patients with an FXIII activity level of less than 30 IU dL^{-1} developed symptoms; 90% of patients with undetectable levels and 46% of patients with levels between the lower limit of detection and 29 IU dL^{-1} had grade III bleeding. Further statistical analysis showed that a level of 15 IU dL^{-1} appears to be the cutoff at which the risk of spontaneous bleeding increases significantly.

Acquired Factor XIII Deficiency

As with other coagulation factor deficiencies, patients can develop an acquired as opposed to inherited FXIII deficiency. Acquired FXIII deficiency is much more common than inherited type FXIII deficiency and can be either immune mediated or non–immune mediated. Non–immune-mediated causes include decreased production in the setting of liver failure and bone marrow failure and more likely are part of a broader coagulation deficiency.[13] Immune-mediated deficiency causes deficiency in the enzyme usually due to an autoantibody binding to plasma FXIII and interfering with its normal function.

One review of 93 cases of immune-mediated FXIII deficiency found that nearly half did not have an identifiable associated cause, with identified causes including malignancy and autoimmune disorders, the former of which were identified in another case report as well.[14] In this same review it was found that 86% of the patients they analyzed had grade III bleeding, suggesting this is a more severe phenotype then congenital FXIII deficiency.[15]

DIAGNOSIS

Patients with FXIII deficiency have normal standard laboratory coagulation tests, such as platelet count, fibrinogen level, bleeding time, prothrombin time, and activated partial thromboplastin time. Diagnosis is made based on clinical presentation, which may include unexplained delayed bleeding or miscarriage, as discussed previously, followed by obtaining a quantitative functional FXIII activity assay. Most patients diagnosed following a bleeding episode have factor levels of less than 30%, whereas those with factor levels of greater than 30% are more likely to remain asymptomatic and be diagnosed only due to family history.[12] If plasma FXIII activity is decreased, the subtype of FXIII deficiency has to be established by either using measurement of FXIII-A and FXIII-B antigen concentration in the plasma or measurement of FXIII activity and FXIII-A antigen in platelet lysate. The antigenic assay easily is automated, allowing ease of performance and, in the authors' institution, is seen to correlate well with the functional measure, especially in the critical 0% to 30% range (**Fig. 1**).

Detection of molecular genetic defects can be performed in patients with suspected hereditary FXIII deficiency. In patients with suspected autoantibodies against FXIII subunits, a mixing study for the detection of neutralizing antibodies against FXIII-A or binding assays for the detection non-neutralizing antibodies against FXIII-A and FXIII-B can be used.[16]

The first case of FXIII deficiency was detected by an abnormal urea clot lysis test. The clot solubility test is only sensitive at a very low levels of FXIII (zero or very close to zero) and the test is normal if the FXIII levels rises to 1% to 3%. Also, clot lysis assays can be falsely normal due to sample handling or other factor level changes like elevated fibrinogen levels.

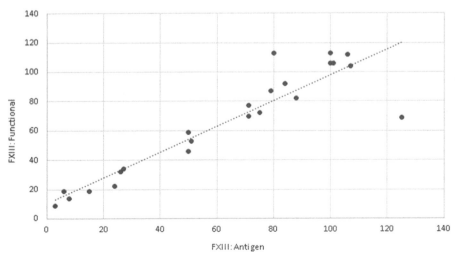

Fig. 1. Correlation of antigen assay and functional measure of FXIII activity.

TREATMENT

Current therapies for patients with FXIII deficiency include recombinant $FXIII-A_2$ for patients with A subunit deficiency or plasma-derived FXIII concentrate for patients with either subunit A or subunit B deficiency. Patients may receive prophylaxis and/or therapeutic replacement of FXIII. When these therapies are not available, various blood products, such as fresh frozen plasma (FFP) and cryoprecipitate, may be used, although some experts prefer cryoprecipitate. The use of FXIII concentrates (plasma derived or recombinant) is recommended when available given decreased volume of transfusions, lower risk of transfusion associated toxicity, and more precise dosing.[17]

Plasma-derived FXIII, a concentrate of FXIII from pooled patient plasma, first was used in the 1980s and became available as a commercial product in Europe in 1993.[18,19] Although there remains some risk of transfusion-associated toxicities, the dosing and level of FXIII are more consistent than FFP and cryoprecipitate. Compared with recombinant FXIII (rFXIII), plasma-derived FXIII contains both A and B subunits, and, for this reason, patients with the rarer B subunit deficiencies should be treated with plasma-derived FXIII as opposed to rFXIII. Although there is a theoretic risk of antibody development to plasma-d,erived FXIII concentrate over time, unlike hemophilia A and hemophilia B this appears to be a rare phenomenon.[20] rFXIII is available and it reported to be safe and effective as a possible alternative plan for FXIII-deficient patients.[21]

Recommendations for the different clinical scenarios associated with FXIII deficiency are reviewed: prophylactic dosing to prevent spontaneous bleeding, preoperative dosing, posttrauma dosing, and preconception and peripartum dosing to prevent miscarriage. These are outlined in **Table 2** as well. There is one major formulation of plasma-derived FXIII concentrate which is produced by CSL Behring and approved as Fibrogammin P in the United States and Corifact in Europe.

Prophylactic

Factor activity levels usually correlate with risk and severity of bleeding in patients with FXIII deficiency. Patients with undetectable FXIII levels are at high risk for spontaneous bleeding, and this risk may persist up to levels as high as 15%.[12] Due to its long half-life (5–11 days), FXIII is an ideal candidate for prophylactic administration due to the ability to administer doses on a relatively infrequent basis.[3] Guidelines from the United Kingdom Haemophilia Centre Doctors' Organisation in 2004 recommended prophylactic dosing of all patients with undetectable factor levels due to the high incidence of potentially fatal intracranial bleeding. They also recommended consideration of prophylactic dosing for patients with levels less than 4%, even in some patients with levels above this range with history of bleeding.[22] The choice of these cutoff values was driven by laboratory data that showed abnormal clotting at levels less than 5% and prior clinical data that seemed to indicate the highest risk of spontaneous bleeding at undetectable levels.[23]

In 2012, a prospective, multicenter, open-label study that was conducted in 41 patients with congenital FXIII deficiency was published, showing benefit of prophylactic dosing.[19] In this study, participants were administered an initial dose of 40 IU/kg every 4 weeks, with dosing adjusted to maintain a trough FXIII activity level of 5% to 20%. Most patients already were on prophylactic FXIII replacement at the time of study initiation with no baseline FXIII activity level required for inclusion in the study. During the 12-month study period, no patients reported spontaneous bleeding while on prophylactic dosing.

Table 2 Treatment of factor XIII deficiency			
	Indication	**Target Level**	**Replacement**
Prophylactic	Baseline levels <5% or any baseline level with history of spontaneous bleeding	≥5%[a] or level at which there is no spontaneous bleeding	Recombinant FXIII-A$_2$ 35 U/kg every 4wk with goal trough level of ≥10% FXIII concentrate 40 U/kg every 4wk, adjust dose by ± 5U/kg dose to maintain trough 5%–20%
Peripartum	All women with history of factor XIII deficiency	>10% peripartum, >30% during labor	Recombinant FXIII-A$_2$ Not specifically studied in this scenario, manufacturer dosing is only for prophylactic setting. FXIII concentrate 1. 250 U per wk through 23-wk goal >10% activity level; then 2. 500 U every wk thereafter to maintain levels above 10% 3. An extra dose of 1000 U prior to labor may be necessary to increase activity level to >30%.
Preoperative	All surgical procedures, although might not be necessary in minor procedures for patients already on prophylactic dosing	Minimum >5% but possibly >50% for major procedures	Recombinant FXIII-A$_2$ Not specifically studied in this scenario; manufacturer dosing is only for prophylactic setting. FXIII concentrate Option 1: 10–20 U/kg for goal >5% preoperatively Option 2: 25–40 U/kg for goal >50% preoperatively
Posttraumatic/ therapeutic	After any clinical episode of bleeding	Minimum >5% but possibly >30%	Recombinant FXIII-A$_2$ Not specifically studied in this scenario; manufacturer dosing is only for prophylactic setting. FXIII concentrate 10–20 U/kg, goal >5% but perhaps upwards of >30% to achieve hemostasis

[a] Possible indication for maintaining levels ≥15%.

More recent data suggest that higher doses of prophylactic FXIII concentrate for neonates may reduce bleeding without any associated complications.[5] In a study from Iran on neonates with diagnosed FXIII deficiency, 17 patients were given a standard dose of Fibrogammin (10–26 IU/kg) whereas 17 other patients received a higher dose of between 60 IU/kg and 80 IU/kg (a complete ampule of the medication was given so as to not waste medication, which led to the variation in dose based on the patient's weight). They then were followed for 3 years, with lower rates of bleeding in the group who received higher doses of Fibrogammin, without any associated thrombotic complications.

Also, in 2012, the first phase 3 study of rFXIIIa was published[21]; 41 patients received monthly (28 d $\pm$ 2 d) doses of 35 IU/kg of rFXIII. There was no prespecified baseline FXIII activity level for inclusion and patients were compared with historic controls. There were no episodes of spontaneous bleeding during the study period among patients receiving the prophylactic rFXIII.

Peripartum

Dosing of FXIII surrounding pregnancy largely is based on case reports and case series. Although patients with FXIII deficiency may be able to bring a pregnancy to term without replacement therapy, there is significant risk for recurrent miscarriage without replacement. In a review of cases, it appears that the risk for miscarriage begins as early as 5 weeks' to 6 weeks' gestation; therefore, starting factor replacement as early in pregnancy as possible is important if a patient is not already on long-term replacement therapy.[10] The optimal dose and factor activity level are poorly defined. As discussed previously, the role and mechanism by which FXIII may lead to pregnancy loss likely are multifactorial; however, it does appear that bleeding plays a role in this process. For this reason, some investigators suggest maintaining a FXIII activity level of greater than 10% similar to recommendations surrounding minor bleeding. During labor, however, the recommendation is to increase this goal to greater than 20% or even 30% due to the higher risk of bleeding.

Even though FXIII concentrate has a long half-life, it appears that the half-life or circulating FXIII shortens as pregnancy progresses, to as little as 1.6 days; therefore, more frequent dosing may be required.[24] Some experts suggest a non–weight-based flat dose of 250 IU of FXIII concentrate once a week through 23 weeks' gestation followed by 500 IU once a week thereafter to maintain levels above 10%. An extra dose of 1000 IU prior to labor may be necessary to increase activity level to greater than 30%.[10] Alternatively, a less aggressive approach has been offered at a dose of 10-IU/kg of plasma-derived FXIII concentrate every 2 weeks during pregnancy.[5]

No evidence-based clinical practice guidelines currently are available to guide prophylactic dosing of high-risk newborn infants. There may be circumstances based on prenatal genetic screening in high-risk communities or families with previously diagnosed children, where newborn infants have a significantly increased possibility of being diagnosed with FXIII deficiency. Given the possibility of life-threatening or life-altering intracranial bleeding in the postpartum period, it may be prudent that newborns requiring testing at the time of birth be treated prophylactically while results are pending.

Preoperative

There is no standard preoperative dosing of FXIII to prevent intraoperative or postoperative bleeding. Evidence for dosing recommendations come from expert opinion and small case series. Guidelines from the United Kingdom Haemophilia Centre Doctors' Organisation in 2004 recommended doses of 10 U/kg to 20 U/kg of plasma-derived FXIII concentrate immediately before surgery, with the goal of keeping FXIII levels "in the normal range" for 5 days postoperatively or until the surgical wound has healed.[22] Normal levels based on population studies are noted to be anywhere between 53.2 IU/dL to 152 IU/dL. The same recommendations were offered by Mannucci and colleagues,[17] recommending 10 U/kg to 20 U/kg prior to major or minor surgery, with a target goal of FXIII activity level of greater than 5%.

Some other single-institution series have reported perioperative and postoperative bleeding, with FXIII levels as high as 40%, and they recommend higher doses to maintain FXIII levels of greater than 50%.[25] This was achieved through tailored dosing, using baseline FXIII activity levels, of FXIII concentrate at doses of 25 U/kg to 40 U/kg.

Some patients may not require additional FXIII prior to minor surgical intervention if they already are maintained on prophylactic FXIII replacement. In one trial, among patients who received prophylactic rFXIII-A_2 at a dose of 35 IU/kg every 28 days $\pm$ 2 days, there were 12 minor surgical procedures performed on 9 patients. In these patients there was no requirement for further preoperative dosing. Although 8 of the 12 procedures were performed within 7 days of the last scheduled dose of factor replacement, 4 were performed beyond 10 days from the last dose up to 21 days. None of the surgical procedures was associated with unexpected blood loos or surgical complications related to their deficiency or treatment.[26]

Therapeutic

Similar to preoperative guidance, the United Kingdom Haemophilia Centre Doctors' Organisation in 2004 recommended doses of 10 U/kg to 20 U/kg of plasma-derived FXIII concentrate in the setting of an acute hemorrhage, with the goal of keeping levels "in the normal range" until there is no further bleeding.[22] Other guidelines recommend targeting trough levels of 30% in the setting of an acute bleed, which is based on previously reported data that patients with levels greater than 30% are less likely to develop bleeding.[6,12] Like other bleeding disorders, treatment should be prompt and initiated upon arrival to prevent further complications.

SUMMARY

FXIII deficiency is a rare autosomal recessive bleeding disorder affecting approximately 1 in 2 million people. Patients with FXIII deficiency are at a significant risk for severe bleeding, especially when levels drop below 5%, but possibly at even higher levels of FXIII activity. Prophylactic therapy is effective at preventing severe spontaneous bleeding and also can be effectively employed to allow for safe surgical intervention.

FXIII deficiency also is uniquely associated with fetal loss. Women should begin replacement therapy prior to or as early in pregnancy as possible aiming for an FXIII trough of greater than 10% during the course of pregnancy and perhaps as high as 30% or more at the time of delivery.

CLINICS CARE POINTS

- Most commonly presents as delayed umbilical cord stump bleeding
- Significant risk for CNS bleeding if left untreated, both spontaneous and posttraumatic
- Patients with FXIII activity level less than 5% are at highest risk for spontaneous bleeding, but patients may experience spontaneous bleeding even at higher levels.

- FXIII can be replaced with FFP, cryoprecipitate, FXIII concentrate or rFXIII.
- rFXIII only contains the A subunit and should not be used for patients with a known B subunit mutation.
- Patients may require increased doses preoperatively even if on prophylactic dosing.
- Women should start replacement therapy with a goal activity level of greater than 10% as early in pregnancy as possible.

DISCLOSURE

The authors have no disclosures.

REFERENCES

1. Dorgalaleh A, Naderi M, Shamsizadeh M. Morbidity and mortality in a large number of Iranian patients with severe congenital factor XIII deficiency. Ann Hematol 2016;95(3):451–5.
2. Sharief LA, Kadir RA. Congenital factor XIII deficiency in women: a systematic review of literature. Haemophilia 2013;19(6):e349–57.
3. Hsieh L, Nugent D. Factor XIII deficiency. Haemophilia 2008;14(6):1190–200.
4. Pisano JJFJ, Peyton MP. Cross-link in fibrin polymerized by factor 13: epsilon-(gamma-glutamyl)lysine. Science 1968;160(3830):892–3.
5. Naderi M, Dorgalaleh A, Alizadeh S, et al. Clinical manifestations and management of life-threatening bleeding in the largest group of patients with severe factor XIII deficiency. Int J Hematol 2014;100(5):443–9.
6. Palla R, Shapiro AD. Rare bleeding disorders: diagnosis and treatment. Blood 2015;125(13):2052–61.
7. Anwar R. Factor XIII deficiency. Br J Haematol 1999;107(3):468–84.
8. Bouttefroy S, Meunier S, Milien V, et al. Congenital factor XIII deficiency: comprehensive overview of the FranceCoag cohort. Br J Haematol 2020;188(2):317–20.
9. Koseki-Kuno S, Yamakawa M, Dickneite G, et al. Factor XIII a subunit-deficient mice developed severe uterine bleeding events and subsequent spontaneous miscarriages. Blood 2003;102(13):4410–2.
10. Asahina TKT, Takeuchi K, Kanayama N. Congenital blood coagulation factor XIII deficiency and successful deliveries: a review of the literature. Obstet Gynecol Surv 2007;62(4):255–60.
11. Peyvandi F, Palla R, Menegatti M, et al. Coagulation factor activity and clinical bleeding severity in rare bleeding disorders: results from the European Network of Rare Bleeding Disorders. J Thromb Haemost 2012;10(4):615–21.
12. Menegatti M, Palla R, Boscarino M, et al. Minimal factor XIII activity level to prevent major spontaneous bleeds. J Thromb Haemost 2017;15(9):1728–36.
13. Yan MTS, Rydz N, Goodyear D, et al. Acquired factor XIII deficiency: a review. Transfus Apher Sci 2018;57(6):724–30.
14. Nixon CPPE, Guertin CA, Stevenson RL, et al. Acquired Factor XIII inhibitor associated with mantle cell lymphoma. Transfusion 2017;57(3):694–9.
15. Ichinose A, Japanese Collaborative Research Group on AH. Autoimmune acquired factor XIII deficiency due to anti-factor XIII/13 antibodies: a summary of 93 patients. Blood Rev 2017;31(1):37–45.
16. Kohler HP, Seitz R, Ariens RA, et al. Factor XIII and fibrinogen SSC subcommittee of the ISTH. Diagnosis and classification of factor XIII deficiencies. J Thromb Haemost 2011;9(7):1404–6.

17. Mannucci PM, Duga S, Peyvandi F. Recessively inherited coagulation disorders. Blood 2004;104(5):1243–52.

18. Winkelman L, Haddon ME, Evans DR, et al. A pasteurized concentrate of human plasma factor XIII for therapeutic use. Thromb Haemost 1986;55:402–5.

19. Nugent D. Corifact™/Fibrogammin® P in the prophylactic treatment of hereditary factor XIII deficiency: results of a prospective, multicenter, open-label study. Thromb Res 2012;130:S12–4.

20. Solomon C, Fries D, Pendrak I, et al. Safety of factor XIII concentrate: analysis of more than 20 years of pharmacovigilance data. Transfus Med Hemother 2016; 43(5):365–73.

21. Inbal A, Oldenburg J, Carcao M, et al. Recombinant factor XIII: a safe and novel treatment for congenital factor XIII deficiency. Blood 2012;119(22):5111–7.

22. Bolton-Maggs PH, Perry DJ, Chalmers EA, et al. The rare coagulation disorders– review with guidelines for management from the United Kingdom Haemophilia Centre Doctors' Organisation. Haemophilia 2004;10(5):593–628.

23. Jennings I, Woods TA, Preston FE, et al. Problems relating to the laboratory diag- nosis of factor XIII deficiency: a UK NEQAS study. J Thromb Haemost 2003;1(12): 2603–8.

24. Asahina T, Kobayashi T, Okada Y, et al. Maternal blood coagulation factor XIII is associated with the development of cytotrophoblastic shell. Placenta 2000;21(4): 388–93.

25. Janbain M, Nugent DJ, Powell JS, et al. Use of factor XIII (FXIII) concentrate in patients with congenital FXIII deficiency undergoing surgical procedures. Trans- fusion 2014;55(1):45–50.

26. Carcao M, Altisent C, Castaman G, et al. Recombinant FXIII (rFXIII-A2) prophy- laxis prevents bleeding and allows for surgery in patients with congenital FXIII A-subunit deficiency. Thromb Haemost 2018;118(3):451–60.

27. Lak M, Ali Sharifian A, Karimi K, et al. Pattern of symptoms in 93 Iranian patients with severe factor XIII deficiency. J Thromb Haemost 2003;1(8):1852–3.

28. Acharya SS, Dimichele DM. Rare bleeding disorder registry: de®ciencies of fac- tors II, V, VII,X, XIII, ®brinogen and dys®brinogenemias. J Thromb Haemost 2004;2(2):248–56.

29. Ivaskevicius V, Kohler HP, Schroeder V, et al, Study Group. International registry on factor XIII deficiency: a basis formed mostly on European data. Thromb Hae- most 2007;97(6):914–21.

30. Viswabandya A, Baidya S, Nair SC, et al. Correlating clinical manifestations with factor levels in rare bleeding disorders: a report from Southern India. Haemo- philia 2012;18(3):e195–200.

Rare Coagulation Factor Deficiencies (Factors VII, X, V, and II)

Glaivy Batsuli, MD[a,b,]*, Peter Kouides, MD[c]

KEYWORDS

- Rare bleeding disorders • Epistaxis • Factor II • Factor V • Factor VII • Factor X
- Heavy menstrual bleeding

KEY POINTS

- Rare coagulation factor deficiencies, more commonly referred to as rare bleeding disorders (RBD), comprise a rare group of disorders that can result in a variety of bleeding symptoms.
- Abnormalities in clotting times and low plasma factor activity levels help guide the diagnosis of factor II, V, VII, and X deficiencies.
- The most common bleeding manifestations in RBD are epistaxis and heavy menstrual bleeding, although intracranial hemorrhage and umbilical cord bleeding can occur in neonates with severe factor deficiencies.
- The ideal treatment modality for RBD are high-purity, single-factor products for each disorder, but alternative treatment modalities exist for factor II and V deficiencies that lack such a product.

INTRODUCTION

von Willebrand disease, hemophilia A, and hemophilia B account for most inherited coagulation factor deficiencies worldwide. Inherited rare coagulation factor deficiencies, more commonly referred to as rare bleeding disorders (RBD), consist of deficiencies in fibrinogen as well as factors II (FII), V (FV), VII (FVII), X (FX), XI (FXI), XIII (FXIII); combined factor V + VIII deficiency; and vitamin K-dependent coagulation factor deficiency. Inherited RBD represent only 3% to 5% of all inherited deficiencies of coagulation factors. However, individuals with RBD can present with clinically significant bleeding and are at risk of delayed diagnosis or misdiagnosis due to the rare

[a] Aflac Cancer and Blood Disorders Center of Children's Healthcare of Atlanta; [b] Department of Pediatrics, Emory University, Atlanta, GA, USA; [c] Mary M. Gooley Hemophilia Center, Rochester Regional Health, 1415 Portland Avenue, Rochester, NY 14621, USA
* Corresponding author. Emory Children's Center, 2015 Uppergate Drive, Room 410, Atlanta, GA 30322.
E-mail address: gbatsul@emory.edu

Hematol Oncol Clin N Am 35 (2021) 1181–1196
https://doi.org/10.1016/j.hoc.2021.07.010
0889-8588/21/© 2021 Elsevier Inc. All rights reserved.

nature of these disorders.[1] RBD are predominantly inherited in an autosomal recessive pattern and are more common in areas with higher rates of consanguineous marriages. The heterozygous state is usually asymptomatic. This review focuses on deficiencies of coagulation FII, FV, FVII, and FX.

Pathophysiology

Factor II (prothrombin) deficiency: The American physician and biochemist Dr Armand J. Quick[2,3] first described FII deficiency in 1947 after observing prolonged prothrombin times (PT) and low FII activity in 2 unrelated families. Prothrombin is a 72-kDa glycoprotein synthesized in the liver in the presence of vitamin K and circulates as an inactive zymogen in the plasma. Prothrombin is activated into the active enzyme thrombin when cleaved by the activated factor X (FXa)-activated factor V (FVa) prothrombinase complex on the phospholipid-rich surface of platelets. Thrombin is a critical factor in multiple pathways of clot formation through activation of platelet aggregation and clot potentiation by activation of FV, FVIII, and FIX that forms a positive feedback loop resulting in further thrombin generation.[4] Furthermore, thrombin helps to stabilize fibrin clot formation through the activation of FXIII and thrombin activatable fibrinolysis inhibitor (TAFI). Thrombin also plays a role in mechanisms of anticoagulation. Thrombin interacts with endothelial protein thrombomodulin to activate protein C, which in turn inactivates FVa and activated FVIII (FVIIIa) to reduce clot formation. Thrombin regulation is important for preventing excessive clot formation. Serine protease inhibitor (serpin) family members, such as heparin cofactor II and protease nexin I, inhibit the catalytic activity of thrombin.[5] Antithrombin, a glycoprotein produced in the liver, can inhibit thrombin and FXa activity when coupled with heparin.[6]

FV deficiency: Dr Paul Owren first described FV deficiency in a Norwegian woman with severe recurrent epistaxis and heavy menstrual bleeding in 1943.[7] FV is a 330-kDa glycoprotein produced in the liver that circulates in plasma. Approximately 20% of FV is stored in the alpha granules of platelets and can be released at sites of vascular injury with platelet degranulation.[8] FV is activated via proteolytic cleavage by thrombin and FXa. FV plays an important role in the propagation phase of coagulation as a component of the prothrombinase complex. FVa complexes with FXa on a phospholipid surface in the presence of calcium to form the prothrombinase complex that cleaves FII into thrombin.[9] Thrombin bound to thrombomodulin activates protein C, which binds protein S, to inactivate FVa and FVIIIa through proteolytic cleavage.[10]

Factor VII deficiency: FVII is a 50-kDa vitamin K-dependent serine protease produced in the liver. FVII plays a critical role in the initiation of clot formation as part of the extrinsic pathway of the coagulation cascade. Upon endothelial injury, tissue factor (TF) is exposed from the vascular lumen where it can activate FVII into activated FVII (FVIIa) forming a TF/FVIIa complex. The TF/FVIIa complex is able to activate FX into FXa (forming the "extrinsic tenase" complex) and FIX into activated FIX (FIXa).[11] This process ultimately results in thrombin generation and fibrin clot formation. The thrombin generated during this process activates FV and FVIII through a positive feedback loop that propagates fibrin clot formation. A small portion of FVII circulates as the active serine protease FVIIa in the absence of active clot formation, which is unique to FVII; this is important because it is circulating plasma FVIIa that first engages TF at the site of injury. Furthermore, FVII can be proteolytically cleaved and activated by the TF/FVIIa complex, thrombin, FIXa, and FXa. FVIIa is primarily inhibited by the lipoprotein tissue factor pathway inhibitor (TFPI).

FX deficiency: FX is a 59-kDa vitamin K-dependent serine protease synthesized in the liver that plays a key role in coagulation as the first enzyme in the common pathway in the formation of a stable fibrin clot. In 1905, Morawitz identified a factor named *thromboplastin* that interacted with *thrombogen* to form thrombin.[12] In 1955, Duckert and colleagues[13] reported a factor deficiency that was distinct from FVII and FIX deficiencies in patients receiving coumarins. Inherited FX deficiency was later identified by 2 independent groups, each of which described a patient (Prower in the United Kingdom and Stuart in the United States) with a bleeding diathesis that could not be attributed to other known coagulation factors deficiencies. The factor in both patients was subsequently named FX. As with other vitamin K-dependent proteins, FX requires posttranslational carboxylation of 11 glutamic acid (Glu) residues for functional activity.[14,15] Both the extrinsic and intrinsic pathways can lead to FX activation. In the extrinsic pathway, FX activation occurs via formation of the TF/FVIIa complex with calcium ions on a phospholipid surface. In the intrinsic pathway, FX activation occurs when FIXa and its cofactor FVIIIa form the intrinsic tenase complex in the presence of calcium ions on a phospholipid surface. FXa is the most important activator of prothrombin, cleaving prothrombin to generate thrombin through the prothrombinase complex. FXa also activates FV and FVIII and hydrolyzes FVII to FVIIa, completing the FVII-FX feedback loop. FXa also forms a quaternary complex with TF/FVIIa by binding to TFPI, which downregulates the extrinsic pathway to thrombin generation. Antithrombin inactivates FXa by forming a complex that is rapidly cleared from the circulation. The protein Z-dependent protease inhibitor, a serpin, also inactivates FXa. Defects in protein Z lead to increased FXa activity and may increase the risk of thrombosis.[16]

Genetics and Disease Classification

FII deficiency: The *F2* gene is encoded on chromosome 11p11-q12 and consists of 10 exons and 8 introns. Missense mutations represent most of the more than 50 different *F2* gene variants that have been identified in patients with FII deficiency, but splicing, nonsense, and deletion/insertion mutations have been reported.[17] Most individuals with FII deficiency are homozygous for the same *F2* mutation inherited in an autosomal recessive pattern as opposed to compound heterozygotes for 2 separate variants. There are 2 forms of FII deficiency: (1) a quantitative deficiency (type 1 deficiency or hypoprothrombinemia) that is characterized by equal reductions in FII activity and antigen levels and (2) a qualitative deficiency (type 2 deficiency or dysprothrombinemia) characterized by discordance in the FII activity and antigen levels in which individuals have low FII activity but normal/near-normal FII antigen levels. There are no reported cases of living individuals with a complete absence of FII.[18] Moreover, an FII knockout model in mice demonstrated embryonic and neonatal lethality, suggesting that complete absence of FII is incompatible with life.[19,20]

   FV deficiency: The *F5* gene is located on chromosome 1q24.2 consisting of 25 exons. Missense, nonsense, splicing, and insertion/deletion mutations have been reported among 26 *F5* variants identified in FV-deficient patients. Half of the identified mutations are within exon 13, which encodes the B domain of FV, whereas the remaining variants are scattered throughout the A and C domains of the *F5* gene.[21] Most cases of FV deficiency are characterized by a type 1 quantitative deficiency, but 25% of individuals with FV deficiency will have low FV activities and normal FV antigen levels consistent with a type 2 qualitative defect.[17,21] Mouse models of FV deficiency demonstrate abnormal embryonic development and early death due to hemorrhage; however, mice with FV activities less than 1% and presence of cross-reacting material are able to survive the neonatal period.

   FVII deficiency: The *F7* gene is located on chromosome 13q34 and consists of 9 exons. There have been more than 200 *F7* gene variants identified that result in FVII deficiency in an autosomal recessive pattern. Most *F7* mutations are a result of missense mutations (~60%), but nonsense, splicing, and deletion/insertion mutations have also been reported.[18] In contrast to mouse knockout models of FII and FV deficiency, the FVII-deficient knockout mouse model does not result in abnormal embryonic development; however, survival to adulthood is significantly impaired due to death from hemorrhages in the neonatal period.[22]

FX deficiency: The *F10* gene is also located on chromosome 13q34 just downstream from the gene encoding for FVII. Combined FVII and FX deficiency has been reported due to large deletion of the long arm of chromosome 13 and/or partial duplication.[23] The coding sequence for FX is homologous to that of the other vitamin K-dependent proteins and is divided into 8 exons, each of which encodes a specific domain within the protein. Approximately 150 mutations have been identified to date. Most mutations (~75%) like in the other RBD are missense mutations with the remaining genetic abnormalities being deletions, nonsense mutations, and splice site mutations.[24] Although mutations are typically homozygous, combined heterozygous mutations resulting in moderate FX deficiency has also been reported.[24] The FX-deficient knockout model results in partial embryonic lethality and fatal neonatal bleeding.[25]

DISCUSSION
Epidemiology

FII deficiency is one of the rarest inherited RBD accounting for only 1.5% of RBD.[26] FII deficiency has an estimated worldwide prevalence of 1 in 2,000,000.[17] In addition, there seems to be a higher prevalence of FII genetic variants in individuals of Latin/Hispanic origin, and approximately 70% patients with FII deficiency are from areas such as Barcelona, Padua, Segovia, and Puerto Rico.[27,28] Likewise, FV deficiency affects an estimated 1 in 1,000,000 individuals and represents 9% of RBD diagnoses. FVII deficiency is the most common of the RBD affecting 1 in 500,000 individuals and accounting for an estimated 38% of individuals with RBD worldwide.[26] Similar to FV deficiency, FX deficiency has an estimated prevalence of 1 in 500,000 to 1,000,000.[29] Higher rates of RBD have been reported in regions with increased rates of consanguinity such as the Middle East, North Africa, India, and Pakistan.[21]

Laboratory Evaluation

First-tier coagulation testing for RBD includes assessment of the PT and activated partial thromboplastin time (aPTT) (**Fig. 1**). In FII, FV, and FX deficiencies, the PT and aPTT will be prolonged. Isolated PT prolongation is observed in FVII deficiency. If available, PT and/or aPTT mixing studies can be helpful in differentiating a true factor deficiency (ie, observed correction of the mixing time) from a factor inhibitor (ie, persistent PT and/or aPTT prolongation despite mixing).[30] Specific factor activity levels should be performed in the setting of abnormal coagulation studies or a known family history to confirm the diagnosis. FII, FV, FVII, and FX activities are determined by a one-stage PT-based clotting assay. The FVII activity assay uses a thromboplastin reagent. Differences in the sensitivity of thromboplastin reagents can result in variability in the measured FVII activity level. Recombinant human and human-derived thromboplastins are considered the most reliable and are recommended in clinical laboratories.[31] Nevertheless, it is important to consider that a normal PT and aPTT does not rule out a mild factor deficiency. Thus, specific factor levels should be obtained if there is a high index of suspicion for RBD. Factor antigen levels via an immunoassay

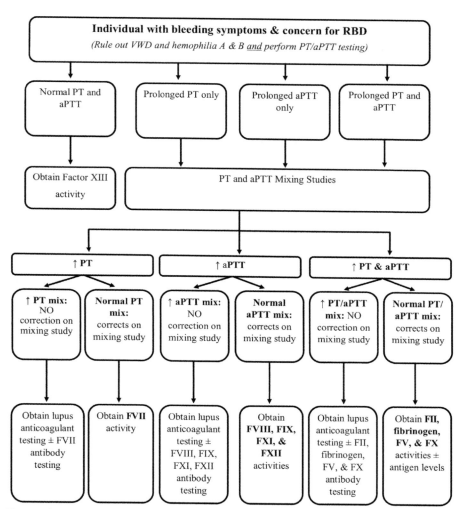

Fig. 1. Algorithm of approach to coagulation testing for RBD. Laboratory testing for an RBD should include evaluation of the complete blood cell count and complete metabolic panel to assess underlying health status and evaluate for cytopenias that could elucidate the cause of bleeding symptoms. Testing for von Willebrand disease and hemophilia A/B should be performed to rule out these more common bleeding disorders. Coagulation testing includes PT and aPTT with mixing studies (if available). Prolonged PT, aPTT, or both PT/aPTT mixing studies help guide testing for specific factor activity levels versus lupus anticoagulant and antibody testing.

can help determine whether an individual possesses a type 1 quantitative versus a type 2 qualitative factor deficiency.

FII, FV, FVII, and FX have reported plasma half-lives of 3 to 4 days, 36 hours, 4 to 6 hours, and 40 to 60 hours, respectively.[17] The half-lives of coagulation factors should be taken into consideration when measuring and interpreting factor activity levels, especially following administration of hemostatic agents such as fresh frozen plasma (FFP), cryoprecipitate, or factor concentrates. A molecular diagnosis of these deficiencies may be helpful in cases of diagnostic uncertainty or in the prenatal setting for families with a known history of RBD and a severe bleeding phenotype; even so, mutation analysis is not required for diagnosis.

Differential Diagnosis

Children with the rare acquired disorder of lupus anticoagulant hypoprothrombinemia syndrome (LAHS) can present with prolonged PT/aPTT and low FII activity similar to inherited FII deficiency. However, patients with LAHS typically present with an acute onset of bleeding symptoms after a viral illness and coagulation studies demonstrate a PT/aPTT mixing study that does not correct, detection of a lupus anticoagulant, and presence of antiprothrombin antibodies. It is important to consider LAHS in the differential diagnoses in individuals younger than 16 years with an acute onset of bleeding, history of a viral prodrome, and prolonged PT/aPTT.[32] Acquired FII, FVII, and FX deficiencies can be observed in the setting of liver disease, disseminated intravascular coagulation, use of vitamin K antagonist warfarin, or vitamin K deficiency. Acquired FV deficiency secondary to an inhibitor has been described primarily in elderly individuals with comorbidities predominantly triggered by antibiotic treatment.[33] There is also report of acquired FV deficiency occurring in a patient with myeloma and amyloidosis.[34] Isolated acquired FVII deficiency can occur in the presence or absence of an FVII inhibitor. Acquired FVII deficiency has been reported in association with severe systemic sepsis, medications, malignancy, aplastic anemia, and posthematopoietic stem cell transplantation.[35,36] Acquired FX deficiency occurs in up to 5% of patients with amyloidosis due to adsorption into splenic amyloid fibrils.[24] There have been reports of acquired FX deficiency with myeloma and other malignancies, infection, and use of sodium valproate. Acquired FX inhibitors have been identified in burns, respiratory infections, and exposure to topical thrombin.[37]

Classification

Classification into the traditional hemophilia categories of mild, moderate, and severe can be challenging in RBD (**Table 1**). Although low factor activity levels can provide confirmation of diagnosis, factor activity levels do not always correlate with the bleeding phenotype. FII activity levels seem to demonstrate a strong correlation with bleeding severity, although data are limited due to its rarity and low prevalence of individuals with FII deficiency.[38] FII activity levels of 20% to 30% are considered hemostatic, and severe bleeding symptoms have been reported primarily in individuals with FII activities less than 10%.[39] Heterozygotes typically have FII activities between 30% and 60% compared with individuals with normal FII activities of greater than 70%. In contrast, FV deficiency has a weak association between bleeding severity and FV activity.[39] FV activity levels of 15% to 20% are considered hemostatic. Yet, severe bleeding symptoms of hemarthrosis and intracranial hemorrhage (ICH) have been described in FV-deficient individuals with FV activities up to 50%.[40] Heterozygotes are usually asymptomatic and have FV activities of 20% to 60%.[28]

In FVII deficiency, individuals with FVII activities less than 10% are at increased risk of major spontaneous bleeding.[39] FVII activities between 15% and 20% are considered hemostatic, and heterozygotes are usually asymptomatic with FVII activities of 40% to 60%. However, the plasma FVII activity level weakly correlates with bleeding risk, even within the same individual over time. One study of European and Latin American individuals with *F7* variants showed that 19% with heterozygous FVII mutations reported bleeding symptoms.[41] In FX deficiency, individuals with FX activities less than 10% are at increased risk of major spontaneous bleeding and patients with levels

Table 1
Summary of prevalence and bleeding manifestations of rare bleeding disorders factor II, factor V, factor VII, and factor X deficiencies

Factor Deficiency	Disease Prevalence	Percentage of RBD[a]	Bleeding Manifestations	Factor Activity and Disease Severity[b]	Correlation of Factor Activity and Clinical Symptoms
FII	1:2,000,000	1.5%	Mucosal bleeding, soft tissue bleeding, & prolonged bleeding following trauma or surgery	Severe: <1% Moderate: 1%–10% Mild: >10% Heterozygotes: 30%–60% Hemostatic level: 20%–30%	Strong association
FV	1:1,000,000	9%	Mucosal bleeding, soft tissue bleeding, & prolonged bleeding following trauma or surgery	Severe: <1% Moderate: 1%–10% Mild: >10% Heterozygotes: 20%–60% Hemostatic level: 15%–20%	Poor association
FVII	1:500,000	38%	Epistaxis, easy bruising, gum bleeding, hemarthrosis, menorrhagia, & trauma- or surgical-induced bleeding	Severe: <10% Moderate: 10%–20% Mild: >20% Heterozygotes: 40%–60% Hemostatic level: 15%–20%	Poor association
FX	1:500,000–1,000,000	8%	Umbilical cording bleeding, hemarthroses, intracranial hemorrhage, mucosal bleeding, muscle bleeding, & hematomas	Severe: <10% Moderate: 10%–40% Mild: >40% Heterozygotes: ~ 50% Hemostatic level: 15%–20%	Strong association

[a] The World Federation of Hemophilia (WFH) survey and EN-RBD project (1).
[b] Data from (1) Palla R, Peyvandi F, Shapiro AD. Rare bleeding disorders: diagnosis and treatment. Blood 2015; 125(13):2052–61 and (2) Peyvandi F, DiMichele D, Bolton-Maggs PHB, et al. Classification of rare bleeding disorders (RBDs) based on the association between coagulant factor activity and clinical bleeding severity. J Thromb Haemost. 2012;9(9):1938–43.

greater than 40% to 60% are usually asymptomatic or have mild bleeding symptoms.[31]

Clinical Manifestations

The most common bleeding manifestations in FII, FV, FVII, and FX deficiencies are mucocutaneous bleeding (ie, epistaxis and heavy menstrual bleeding) and prolonged bleeding following injury or surgery.[28] Neonates with RBD, particularly individuals with severe FVII and FX deficiencies, can present with umbilical stump bleeding and ICH at birth or shortly thereafter. Central nervous system morbidity in the North American Rare Bleeding Disorder (NARBD) registry was reported in 2% to 22% of these RBD.[28] In FX deficiency, mutations associated with ICH may justify genotyping soon after birth wherein the clinician may consider prophylaxis if present.[42] Hemarthroses, muscle hematomas, gastrointestinal bleeding, and easy bruising have also been reported in these RBD.[31,38] In the NARBD registry, the range of musculoskeletal complications including hemarthrosis and muscle contractures ranged from 7% in FX deficiency, 23% in FV deficiency, to 17% to 18% in FII and FVII deficiencies.[28] Heavy menstrual bleeding is a significant bleeding complication with a reported prevalence of 52% in women and girls with RBD.[43] Women with RBD are also at increased risk of bleeding during pregnancy, delivery, and postpartum and may have an increased risk of fetal loss.[44] Reproductive age issues related to RBD are further discussed later in this review.

Heterozygote carriers regardless of gender are usually asymptomatic, except for heterozygous FV, FVII, and FX carriers, of which a portion have reported bleeding symptoms.[28,40] A study of 128 FX heterozygotes matched with an unaffected family member by gender and age noted that 29.7% had 1 or more bleeding symptom compared with 2.3% of control subjects.[45] The most common symptom was bleeding following an invasive procedure (ie, dental extraction or surgery).

Therapeutic Options

Recommendations by the European Network of Rare Bleeding Disorders (EN-RBD) project advise minimum plasma FII, FV, FVII, and FX activities of greater than 10%, 10%, greater than 20%, and 40%, respectively, as the target factor trough levels to prevent bleeding symptoms.[29] At present, there are no single-factor concentrates commercially available for FII- and FV-deficient individuals. There are dedicated single-factor products for FVII- and FX-deficient individuals. Recommendations for on-demand and prophylactic dosing of factor concentrates of these RBD are outlined in **Table 2**.

FFP and prothrombin complex concentrates (PCCs) are the primary treatment modalities for management of acute bleeding events, surgical hemostasis, and long-term prophylaxis in FII deficiency. PCCs contain various amounts of factors II, VII, IX, and X depending on whether it is a 3-factor PCC (contains FII, FIX, and FX) or a 4-factor PCC (contains FII, FVII, FIX, and FX). In a few countries, a virally inactivated FFP product via solvent/detergent treatment of pooled plasma is available for individuals with RBD.[46] In most countries, FFP is tested for specific viruses but not virally inactivated. When available, solvent/detergent-treated FFP, or other mechanism of viral inactivation, is preferred for treatment in this patient population.

Neither PCCs nor cryoprecipitate contain FV, thus FFP is the mainstay of treatment in FV-deficient patients to increase their FV activity levels. Platelet transfusions have been used in combination with FFP in FV deficiency because a portion of FV is stored in platelet alpha granules, but the risk of platelet alloimmunization must be considered.[47,48]

Table 2
Recommended on-demand and prophylactic treatment of rare bleeding disorders factor II, factor V, factor VII, and factor X deficiencies

Factor Deficiency	Factor Plasma Half-Life	Recommended Factor Trough Levels[a]	On-Demand Treatment	Prophylactic Treatment[b]
FII	3–4 d	>10%	FFP[c] 15–25 mL/kg PCC (3-F or 4-F) 20–40 U/kg	FFP[c] not preferred for prophylaxis PCC (3-F or 4-F) 20–40 U/kg 1 time/wk
FV	36 h	10%	FFP[c] 15–25 mL/kg Platelets: consider transfusion as adjunct therapy to FFP in certain circumstances	FFP[c] 15–20 mL/kg 2 times/wk Platelets are not preferred for prophylaxis
FVII	4–6 h	>20%	FFP[c] not preferred pdFVII concentrate 30–40 U/kg Recombinant FVIIa 15–30 µg/kg	FFP[c] 10–20 mL/kg 2 times/wk pdFVII concentrate 30–40 U/kg 3 times/wk Recombinant FVIIa 15–30 µg/kg 3 times/wk
FX	40–60 h	>40%	FFP[c] 10–20 mL/kg PCC (3-F or 4-F) 20–40 U/kg pd-FX/FIX concentrate 10–20 U/kg pdFX concentrate 25 U/kg	FFP[c] not preferred for prophylaxis PCC (3-F or 4-F) 20–40 U/kg 2 times/wk pd-FX/FIX concentrate 10–20 U/kg 2 times/wk pdFX concentrate 25 U/kg 2 times/wk

Abbreviations: 3-F, 3-factor PCC; 4-F, 4-factor PCC; FFP, fresh frozen plasma; FVIIa, activated factor VII; PCC, prothrombin complex concentrate; pdFVII, plasma-derived FVII concentrate; pdFX, plasma-derived FX concentrate; pdFX/FIX, plasma-derived FX and FIX concentrate.

[a] *Data from* Menegatti M, Peyvandi F. Treatment of rare factor deficiencies other than hemophilia. Blood. 2019;133(5):415–24 and Mumford AD, Ackroyd S, Alikhan R, et al. Guideline for the diagnosis and management of the rare coagulation disorders: a United Kingdom Haemophilia Centre Doctors' Organization guideline on behalf of the British Committee for Standards in Haematology. Br J Haematol. 2014;167(3):304–26.

[b] Factor dose and administration frequency may vary in the pediatric population (especially in children <12 years old) to achieve the recommended factor trough levels in light of increased factor metabolism expected in this population.

[c] Viral inactivated (eg, solvent/detergent-treated) FFP preferred.

Recombinant activated FVII (rFVIIa) is the preferred treatment product in FVII deficiency for severe bleeding symptoms or surgical management. However, rFVIIa infusions administered 2 to 3 times per week for prophylaxis has been used successfully despite the short half-life.[49] In some areas of the world, a plasma-derived FVII concentrate is available as an alternative treatment when rFVIIa is not available. PCCs are not recommended in FVII deficiency due to limited or no FVII.

Historically, FFP or PCCs have been used for replacement therapy in FX deficiency. However since 2015, a high-purity, plasma-derived FX (pdFX) concentrate has been available.[50] Viral inactivation of pdFX includes solvent/detergent treatment, nanofiltration, and terminal heat treatment. A phase 3 pharmacokinetic study of 16 patients with moderate to severe FX deficiency (<5%) using a pdFX dose of 25 IU/kg established a half-life of 29.4 hours and incremental recovery of 2.00 IU/dL suggesting prophylactic dosing of 1 to 2 times per week.[51] In the Ten01 trial, 16 patients were infused 25 IU/kg pdFX for 187 bleeds over a minimum study period of 6 to 24 months.[52] Subjective rating for efficacy was "excellent or good" in 98% of subjects. A small surgical study in 5 patients undergoing 7 surgeries reported 100% efficacy.[53] No major adverse events or onset of inhibitory antibodies have been reported. In neonates and infants, higher dosing of 70 to 80 IU/kg for on-demand treatment and prophylaxis seems necessary.[54] In 9 children with FX less than 5%, there is a recent report of its use successfully for prophylaxis and on-demand treatment with efficacy graded excellent at a pdFX regimen of ~40 IU/kg every 3 days.[55]

Antifibrinolytic drugs ε-aminocaproic acid and tranexamic acid are commonly used and recommended for mild bleeding symptoms such as mucocutaneous bleeding and minor surgical procedures in all RBD.

Reproductive Issues

In general, women and girls with heavy menstrual bleeding have benefited from hormonal therapies including combined oral contraceptives containing estrogen, progestin-only agents, and intrauterine devices as monotherapy or adjunctive therapy with other hemostatic agents, such as antifibrinolytic drugs.[44,56]

FII and FV levels are unchanged and remain stable throughout pregnancy and delivery. FII activity less than 20% is considered insufficient for delivery as antepartum and postpartum hemorrhage has been reported in women with FII activities in this range. Thus, administration of PCC at 20 to 40 IU/kg is advised during labor or before cesarean delivery to achieve 20% to 40% FII activity levels.[38] Similarly, in FV deficiency an FV activity less than 20% is considered insufficient to support a safe delivery and prevent postpartum hemorrhage. FFP administration at 15 to 25 mL/kg to achieve a minimum FV activity of 20% to 40% at time of established labor or before cesarean section is recommended.[38] Subsequent FFP transfusions at 10 mL/kg every 12 hours for a minimum of 3 days to maintain FV activity levels greater than 20% has been reported in the literature.[57]

FVII activity does increase during pregnancy, and women with mild FVII deficiency may achieve hemostatic FVII activity levels that are adequate for delivery. However, women with severe FVII deficiency remain at increased risk for hemorrhage and pregnancy loss with persistently low FVII activity. In one report of more than 90 live births in women with FVII deficiency, FVII replacement was administered in only 32% of births. Postpartum hemorrhage occurred in 13% of deliveries with FVII replacement versus 10% of deliveries without FVII replacement.[58] Given the discrepancy between FVII activity and bleeding phenotype, delivery management of women with FVII deficiency should be decided on a case-by-case basis.[59] One report suggests consideration of rFVIIa infusion at 15 to 30 μg/kg every 4 to 6 hours for a minimum of 3 days in women with a severe bleeding history, FVII activity less than 20% in the third trimester, or before cesarean delivery.[57]

Spiliopoulos and Kadir[60] carried out a systematic review of obstetric and gyneco-logic aspects of FX deficiency in 332 patients. A quarter had heavy menses with 66% requiring blood products. Hemoperitoneum was reported in 2.4% with 6 of 8 requiring surgical intervention and 2 of 6 requiring an oophorectomy. Of 31 pregnan-cies in 19 women with FX deficiency, 30% were preterm births and 38% of the preterm births resulted in neonatal death. Most women who had preterm births were not on FX prophylaxis. Postpartum hemorrhage occurred in 22% of deliveries with one culmi-nating in a hysterectomy. Prophylactic FX infusions via pdFX, PCC, or FFP during pregnancy should be considered if there are systemic bleeding symptoms, vaginal bleeding, retroplacental hematoma, or history of fetal loss. A scheduled or cesarean delivery facilitates coordination of obstetrics, hematology, and hospital pharmacy and should be considered on an individual basis. Factor replacement with pdFX 25 IU/kg, FFP 10 to 15 mL/kg, or PCC 20 to 40 IU/kg should be administered at the onset of labor targeting FX activities of 20% to 40%.[61] Recommendations for management of women with severe FX deficiency through the reproductive years have been pre-sented by Nance and colleagues.[62]

Research

Given the rarity of RBD worldwide, prospective clinical studies evaluating optimal treatment approaches and novel therapies are challenging to perform and thus remain limited. National and international registries such as the EN-RBD,[39] the NARBD regis-try,[28] and United Kingdom Haemophilia Centre Doctors' Organization Registry[38] have proved to be critical resources for advancing knowledge on RBD phenotype, geno-type, and management. For FII and FV deficiencies, no factor-specific concentrates are currently approved for bleeding management. A solvent/detergent-treated plasma-derived FV concentrate in development has been tested using plasma sam-ples from adult patients with FV deficiency.[63] Plasma samples spiked with the FV concentrate demonstrated a linear dose-dependent improvement in standard clotting assays (ie, PT/aPTT), FV activities, FV antigen levels, and thrombin generation profiles. Although this FV concentrate shows great promise, this concentrate is not yet commercially available and further studies evaluating safety and efficacy in individuals with FV deficiency are warranted. Long-acting fusion molecules that seek to extend the short half-life of rFVIIa have been in development and studied preclinically; how-ever, these studies have yet to be investigated or approved in FVII deficiency.[29]

Gene therapy trials have primarily focused on increasing coagulation protein expression in hemophilia A and B; however, expression of the FVII zymogen using a liver-directed adeno-associated virus serotype 8 has been explored in dogs with FVII activity less than 1%.[64] FVII-deficient dogs achieved clinically therapeutic FVII ac-tivity of 15% or more, which was sustained for more than 1 year without evidence of aberrations in prothrombotic markers. However, further studies are warranted.

SUMMARY

RBD consist of a group of inherited bleeding disorders that share similarities in path-ophysiology of disease and clinical presentation but can vary in disease management. Although these disorders affect a small population of individuals worldwide, bleeding symptoms can significantly impact an individual's quality of life and result in adverse bleeding-associated complications. The clinician must remain cognizant that these patients can have the "worst" of both worlds of severe hemophilia and von Willebrand disease in terms of both deep tissue and mucosal bleeding and major obstetric and menstrual bleeding complications. The clinician must also be aware of risk of bleeding in some heterozygotes. Factor replacement remains the primary treatment modality in each of the RBD. Adjuvant therapies such as antifibrinolytics and hormonal therapies in women with heavy menses greatly supplement the management of bleeding symptoms. Further research addressing the RBD that lack a dedicated, high-purity, single-factor product as well as alternative factor replacement and drug development warrant greater attention. Further clinical care and research regarding indications for prophylaxis in general and in the obstetric and gynecologic setting is also needed.

CLINICS CARE POINTS

- RBD can present with a variety of bleeding symptoms including deep tissue and mucosal bleeding that ranges from mild to severe and can present in the neonatal period into adulthood.
- Evaluation of the PT, aPTT, PT/aPTT mixing studies and factor activity and antigen levels are important laboratory studies for establishing RBD diagnosis.
- Molecular testing of factor genes can aid in the diagnosis but are not mandatory for RBD. Certain mutations may correlate with higher risk of severe bleeds, such as ICH, and may suggest the need for early initiation of factor prophylaxis.
- Plasma factor activity levels do not always correlate with the bleeding risk for some of the RBD. Clinical assessment of bleeding is consequently paramount beyond the level itself with treatment appropriate even in cases of "moderate or mild" factor deficiency.
- Routine follow-up by providers with expertise in managing patients with inherited bleeding disorders or at a facility with a dedicated comprehensive care model of care akin to the care of individuals with hemophilia A and B, in addition to obstetric and gynecologic multidisciplinary engagement, is strongly advised to optimize patient care and outcomes over the age spectrum.

DISCLOSURE

G.B. has received honorarium from Bio Products Laboratory, the manufacturer of plasma-derived factor X concentrate. P.K. has no conflicts of interests to declare.

REFERENCES

1. Peyvandi F, Menegatti M. Treatment of rare factor deficiencies in 2016. Hematol Am Soc Hematol Educ Program 2016;2016(1):663–9.
2. Quick AJ. Congenital hypoprothrombinaemia and pseudo-hypoprothrombinaemia. Lancet 1947;2(6472):379–82.
3. Quick AJ, Hussey CV. Hereditary hypoprothrombinaemias. Lancet 1962;1(7222): 173–7.
4. Meeks SL, Abshire TC. Abnormalities of prothrombin: a review of the pathophysiology, diagnosis, and treatment. Haemophilia 2008;14(6):1159–63.
5. Davie EW, Kulman JD. An overview of the structure and function of thrombin. Semin Thromb Hemost 2006;32(Suppl 1):3–15.
6. Girolami A, Cosi E, Ferrari S, et al. New clotting disorders that cast new light on blood coagulation and may play a role in clinical practice. J Thromb Thrombolysis 2017;44(1):71–5.

7. Stormorken H. The discovery of factor V: a tricky clotting factor. J Thromb Haemost 2003;1(2):206–13.

8. Kalafatis M. Coagulation factor V: a plethora of anticoagulant molecules. Curr Opin Hematol 2005;12(2):141–8.

9. Mann KG, Nesheim ME, Church WR, et al. Surface-dependent reactions of the vitamin K-dependent enzyme complexes. Blood 1990;76(1):1–16.

10. Tabibian S, Shiravand Y, Shams M, et al. A Comprehensive Overview of Coagulation Factor V and Congenital Factor V Deficiency. Semin Thromb Hemost 2019; 45(5):523–43.

11. Spronk HM, de Jong AM, Crijns HJ, et al. Pleiotropic effects of factor Xa and thrombin: what to expect from novel anticoagulants. Cardiovasc Res 2014; 101(3):344–51.

12. Girolami A, Cosi E, Sambado L, et al. Complex history of the discovery and characterization of congenital factor X deficiency. Semin Thromb Hemost 2015;41(4): 359–65.

13. Duckert F, Fluckiger P, Matter M, et al. Clotting factor X; physiologic and physicochemical properties. Proc Soc Exp Biol Med Soc Exp Biol Med (New York, NY) 1955;90(1):17–22.

14. Telfer TP, Denson KW, Wright DR. A new coagulation defect. Br J Haematol 1956; 2(3):308–16.

15. Hougie C, Barrow EM, Graham JB. Stuart clotting defect. I. Segregation of an hereditary hemorrhagic state from the heterogeneous group heretofore called stable factor (SPCA, proconvertin, factor VII) deficiency. J Clin Invest 1957;36(3): 485–96.

16. Razzari C, Martinelli I, Bucciarelli P, et al. Polymorphisms of the protein Z-dependent protease inhibitor (ZPI) gene and the risk of venous thromboembolism. Thromb Haemost 2006;95(5):909–10.

17. Mannucci PM, Duga S, Peyvandi F. Recessively inherited coagulation disorders. Blood 2004;104(5):1243–52.

18. Peyvandi F, Kunicki T, Lillicrap D. Genetic sequence analysis of inherited bleeding diseases. Blood 2013;122(20):3423–31.

19. Sun WY, Witte DP, Degen JL, et al. Prothrombin deficiency results in embryonic and neonatal lethality in mice. Proc Natl Acad Sci U S A 1998;95(13):7597–602.

20. Sun WY, Coleman MJ, Witte DP, et al. Rescue of prothrombin-deficiency by transgene expression in mice. Thromb Haemost 2002;88(6):984–91.

21. Peyvandi F, Duga S, Akhavan S, et al. Rare coagulation deficiencies. Haemophilia 2002;8(3):308–21.

22. Rosen ED, Chan JC, Idusogie E, et al. Mice lacking factor VII develop normally but suffer fatal perinatal bleeding. Nature 1997;390(6657):290–4.

23. Hutchins K, Rajpurkar M, Stockton DW, et al. Factor VII and factor X deficiency in a child with a chromosome 13q duplication and deletion. Haemophilia 2021; 27(1):e127–8.

24. Mitchell M, Gattens M, Kavakli K, et al. Genotype analysis and identification of novel mutations in a multicentre cohort of patients with hereditary factor X deficiency. Blood Coagul Fibrinolysis 2019;30(1):34–41.

25. Dewerchin M, Liang Z, Moons L, et al. Blood coagulation factor X deficiency causes partial embryonic lethality and fatal neonatal bleeding in mice. Thromb Haemost 2000;83(2):185–90.

26. Palla R, Peyvandi F, Shapiro AD. Rare bleeding disorders: diagnosis and treatment. Blood 2015;125(13):2052–61.

27. Lancellotti S, Basso M, De Cristofaro R. Congenital prothrombin deficiency: an update. Semin Thromb Hemost 2013;39(6):596–606.

28. Acharya SS, Coughlin A, Dimichele DM. Rare Bleeding Disorder Registry: deficiencies of factors II, V, VII, X, XIII, fibrinogen and dysfibrinogenemias. J Thromb Haemost 2004;2(2):248–56.

29. Menegatti M, Peyvandi F. Treatment of rare factor deficiencies other than hemophilia. Blood 2019;133(5):415–24.

30. Acharya SS. Rare bleeding disorders in children: identification and primary care management. Pediatrics 2013;132(5):882–92.

31. Peyvandi F, Di Michele D, Bolton-Maggs PH, et al. Classification of rare bleeding disorders (RBDs) based on the association between coagulant factor activity and clinical bleeding severity. J Thromb Haemost 2012;10(9):1938–43.

32. Sarker T, Roy S, Hollon W, et al. Lupus anticoagulant acquired hypoprothrombinemia syndrome in childhood: two distinct patterns and review of the literature. Haemophilia 2015;21(6):754–60.

33. Goulenok T, Vasco C, Faille D, et al. Acquired factor V inhibitor: a nation-wide study of 38 patients. Br J Haematol 2021;192(5):892–9.

34. Quek JKS, Wong WH, Tan CW, et al. Acquired factor V deficiency in a patient with myeloma and amyloidosis. Thromb Res 2018;164:1–3.

35. Mulliez SM, Devreese KM. Isolated acquired factor VII deficiency: review of the literature. Acta clinica Belgica 2016;71(2):63–70.

36. Girolami A, Santarossa C, Cosi E, et al. Acquired Isolated FVII Deficiency: An Underestimated and Potentially Important Laboratory Finding. Clin Appl Thromb Hemost 2016;22(8):705–11.

37. Lee G, Duan-Porter W, Metjian AD. Acquired, non-amyloid related factor X deficiency: review of the literature. Haemophilia 2012;18(5):655–63.

38. Mumford AD, Ackroyd S, Alikhan R, et al. Guideline for the diagnosis and management of the rare coagulation disorders: a United Kingdom Haemophilia Centre Doctors' Organization guideline on behalf of the British Committee for Standards in Haematology. Br J Haematol 2014;167(3):304–26.

39. Peyvandi F, Palla R, Menegatti M, et al. Coagulation factor activity and clinical bleeding severity in rare bleeding disorders: results from the European Network of Rare Bleeding Disorders. J Thromb Haemost 2012;10(4):615–21.

40. Delev D, Pavlova A, Heinz S, et al. Factor 5 mutation profile in German patients with homozygous and heterozygous factor V deficiency. Haemophilia 2009; 15(5):1143–53.

41. Herrmann FH, Wulff K, Auerswald G, et al. Factor VII deficiency: clinical manifestation of 717 subjects from Europe and Latin America with mutations in the factor 7 gene. Haemophilia 2009;15(1):267–80.

42. Diesch T, von der Weid NX, Schifferli A, et al. Intracranial Hemorrhage as the First Manifestation of Severe Congenital Factor X Deficiency in a 20-Month-Old Male: Case Report and Review of the Literature. Pediatr Blood Cancer 2016;63(7): 1300–4.

43. Siboni SM, Spreafico M, Calò L, et al. Gynaecological and obstetrical problems in women with different bleeding disorders. Haemophilia 2009;15(6):1291–9.

44. Peyvandi F, Garagiola I, Menegatti M. Gynecological and obstetrical manifestations of inherited bleeding disorders in women. J Thromb Haemost 2011; 9(Suppl 1):236–45.

45. Girolami A, Cosi E, Santarossa C, et al. Prevalence of bleeding manifestations in 128 heterozygotes for Factor X deficiency, mainly for FX Friuli, matched versus

128 unaffected family members, during a long sequential observation period (23.5 years). Eur J Haematol 2016;97(6):547–53.

46. Solheim BG, Seghatchian J. Update on pathogen reduction technology for therapeutic plasma: an overview. Transfus Apher Sci 2006;35(1):83–90.

47. Drzymalski DM, Elsayes AH, Ward KR, et al. Platelet transfusion as treatment for factor V deficiency in the parturient: a case report. Transfusion (Paris) 2019;59(7): 2234–7.

48. Di Paola J, Nugent D, Young G. Current therapy for rare factor deficiencies. Haemophilia 2001;7(Suppl 1):16–22.

49. Napolitano M, Giansily-Blaizot M, Dolce A, et al. Prophylaxis in congenital factor VII deficiency: indications, efficacy and safety. Results from the Seven Treatment Evaluation Registry (STER). Haematologica 2013;98(4):538–44.

50. Shapiro A. Plasma-derived human factor X concentrate for on-demand and perioperative treatment in factor X-deficient patients: pharmacology, pharmacokinetics, efficacy, and safety. Expert Opin Drug Metab Toxicol 2017;13(1): 97–104.

51. Austin SK, Brindley C, Kavakli K, et al. Pharmacokinetics of a high-purity plasma-derived factor X concentrate in subjects with moderate or severe hereditary factor X deficiency. Haemophilia 2016;22(3):426–32.

52. Austin SK, Kavakli K, Norton M, et al. Efficacy, safety and pharmacokinetics of a new high-purity factor X concentrate in subjects with hereditary factor X deficiency. Haemophilia 2016;22(3):419–25.

53. Escobar MA, Auerswald G, Austin S, et al. Experience of a new high-purity factor X concentrate in subjects with hereditary factor X deficiency undergoing surgery. Haemophilia 2016;22(5):713–20.

54. Zimowski KL, McGuinn CE, Abajas YL, et al. Use of plasma-derived factor X concentrate in neonates and infants with congenital factor X deficiency. J Thromb Haemost 2020;18(10):2551–6.

55. Liesner R, Akanezi C, Norton M, et al. Prophylactic treatment of bleeding episodes in children <12 years with moderate to severe hereditary factor X deficiency (FXD): Efficacy and safety of a high-purity plasma-derived factor X (pdFX) concentrate. Haemophilia 2018;24(6):941–9.

56. Lee CA, Chi C, Pavord SR, et al. The obstetric and gynaecological management of women with inherited bleeding disorders–review with guidelines produced by a taskforce of UK Haemophilia Centre Doctors' Organization. Haemophilia 2006; 12(4):301–36.

57. Girolami A, Scandellari R, Lombardi AM, et al. Pregnancy and oral contraceptives in factor V deficiency: a study of 22 patients (five homozygotes and 17 heterozygotes) and review of the literature. Haemophilia 2005;11(1):26–30.

58. Baumann Kreuziger LM, Morton CT, Reding MT. Is prophylaxis required for delivery in women with factor VII deficiency? Haemophilia 2013;19(6):827–32.

59. Lee EJ, Burey L, Abramovitz S, et al. Management of pregnancy in women with factor VII deficiency: A case series. Haemophilia 2020;26(4):652–6.

60. Spiliopoulos D, Kadir RA. Congenital Factor X deficiency in women: A systematic review of the literature. Haemophilia 2019;25(2):195–204.

61. Kulkarni R, James AH, Norton M, et al. Efficacy, safety and pharmacokinetics of a new high-purity factor X concentrate in women and girls with hereditary factor X deficiency. J Thromb Haemost 2018;16(5):849–57.

62. Nance D, Josephson NC, Paulyson-Nunez K, et al. Factor X deficiency and pregnancy: preconception counselling and therapeutic options. Haemophilia 2012; 18(3):e277–85.

63. Bulato C, Novembrino C, Anzoletti MB, et al. "In vitro" correction of the severe factor V deficiency-related coagulopathy by a novel plasma-derived factor V concentrate. Haemophilia 2018;24(4):648–56.

64. Marcos-Contreras OA, Smith SM, Bellinger DA, et al. Sustained correction of FVII deficiency in dogs using AAV-mediated expression of zymogen FVII. Blood 2016; 127(5):565–71.

Disorders of Fibrinogen and Fibrinolysis

Jori E. May, MD[a], Alisa S. Wolberg, PhD[b], Ming Yeong Lim, MBBChir[c],*

KEYWORDS

- Coagulation • Hemostasis • Fibrinogen • Afibrinogenemia • Hypofibrinogenemia
- Dysfibrinogenemia • Fibrinolysis • D-dimer

KEY POINTS

- Disorders in fibrinogen concentration and/or function can increase the risk of bleeding and/or thrombosis.
- Depending on the clinical situation, fibrinogen concentrates may be used to achieve hemostatic control in fibrinogen disorders.
- Disorders of fibrinolysis can be congenital or acquired secondary to various clinical situations including trauma, malignancy, or sepsis.
- Antifibrinolytics are a mainstay of treatment for hyperfibrinolysis.

BACKGROUND

Fibrinogen is a large (340 kDa) hexameric glycoprotein expressed by hepatocytes.[1] Fibrinogen is encoded by 3 different genes (*FGA*, *FGB*, and *FGG*) and assembled as a dimer of trimers, with each half consisting of 3 polypeptide chains known as Aα, Bβ, and γ (**Fig. 1**). These chains are arranged with N-termini in the center of the molecule and C-termini extending outward, and are held together by disulfide bonds. Once secreted, fibrinogen circulates in plasma at a concentration of 200 to 400 mg/dL, with a half-life of 3 to 4 days.[1] As an acute-phase protein, fibrinogen levels in circulation may increase 2- to 4-fold during an inflammatory response.

Fibrinogen plays an important role in both primary and secondary hemostasis. During primary hemostasis, the carboxy-terminal end of the γ chains bind to

a Division of Hematology/Oncology, University of Alabama at Birmingham, 1720 2nd Avenue South, NP 2503, Birmingham, AL 35294, USA; b UNC Department of Pathology and Laboratory Medicine, UNC Blood Research Center, 8018A Mary Ellen Jones Building, CB7035, Chapel Hill, NC 27599-7035, USA; c Department of Internal Medicine, Division of Hematology and Hematologic Malignancies, University of Utah, 2000 Circle Hope Drive, Room 4126, Salt Lake City, UT 84112, USA
* Corresponding author.
E-mail address: ming.lim@hsc.utah.edu

Hematol Oncol Clin N Am 35 (2021) 1197–1217
https://doi.org/10.1016/j.hoc.2021.07.011
0889-8588/21/© 2021 Elsevier Inc. All rights reserved.

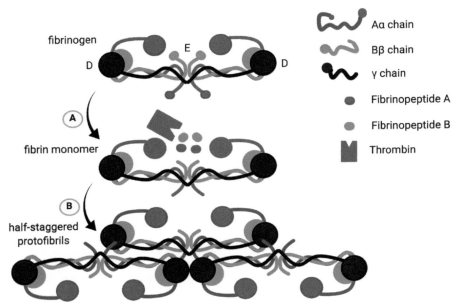

Fig. 1. Conversion of fibrinogen to fibrin. (*A*) Thrombin cleaves fibrinopeptides on the N-termini of the Aα and Bβ chains, resulting in fibrin monomers. (*B*) Polymerization of the fibrin monomers occurs between the newly exposed knobs in the N-termini of the α and β chains (E-domain) of one fibrin monomer and the C-terminal regions of the γ and β chain (in the D-domain) of another fibrin monomer in a half-staggered pattern to form fibrin protofibrils.

glycoprotein IIb–IIIa (integrin αIIbβ3) on the surface of activated platelets, leading to platelet aggregation and the formation of a platelet "plug" at the site of tissue injury.[2] In secondary hemostasis, fibrinogen is converted into fibrin in a stepwise manner.[1,3] First, thrombin cleaves fibrinopeptides on the N-termini of the Aα and Bβ chains, producing fibrin monomers (see **Fig. 1**A). Next, polymerization of the fibrin monomers occurs via interactions between the newly exposed N-terminal knobs of the α and β chains (E-domain) of one fibrin monomer and pockets in the C-terminal domains of the γ and β chains (D-domain) of another fibrin monomer. This process results in a half-staggered conformation, forming fibrin protofibrils (see **Fig. 1**B). Protofibrils undergo lateral aggregation to produce fibers, which branch to form the fibrin network. The fibrin network becomes crosslinked by activated factor XIII (FXIIIa), which catalyzes the formation of intermolecular ε-N-(γ-glutamyl)-lysyl crosslinks that stabilize and strengthen the structural integrity of the fibrin clot.[4]

A physiologic variant of fibrinogen, fibrinogen γ' (γA/γ'), occurs due to alternative splicing of the γ-chain mRNA and constitutes about 8% to 15% of overall fibrinogen in plasma.[5] Fibrinogen γ' has a complex modulatory effect on thrombin activity. Fibrinogen γ' binds to thrombin with high affinity, and sequesters thrombin into the fibrin clot, thus reducing the availability of thrombin in plasma (an antithrombin-like activity of fibrinogen γ'). Conversely, the sequestration of thrombin into the fibrin clot protects thrombin against inhibition by antithrombin and heparin.[6,7] Fibrinogen γ' can also influence fibrin clot architecture. Fibers produced with fibrinogen γ' have reduced protofibril packing and less compact structures, and fibrin clots containing the γ' isoform are resistant to lysis.[8–10]

During the process leading to fibrin dissolution (fibrinolysis), plasminogen is activated to plasmin by one of the two serine proteases, tPA (tissue-type plasminogen activator) or uPA (urokinase-type plasminogen activator) (**Fig. 2**).[11] The binding of tPA and plasminogen to lysine residues on fibrin facilitates plasmin generation.[12] Plasmin then cleaves the fibrin fibers, releasing fibrin degradation products (FDPs), including D-dimer.

The fibrinolytic system is inhibited by serpins, including plasminogen activator inhibitor-1 (PAI-1) and α_2-antiplasmin (α_2AP), and a nonserpin inhibitor, thrombin-activated fibrinolysis inhibitor (TAFI) (see **Fig. 2**).[11] PAI-1 is released in high concentrations by endothelial cells, monocytes, hepatocytes, and adipocytes, and rapidly inhibits both tPA and uPA, resulting in their short half-lives in circulation (approximately 4–8 minutes).[13] α_2AP is synthesized by hepatocytes and binds to and inactivates plasmin. When plasmin is bound to fibrin, it is protected from inactivation by α_2AP, thus highlighting complex contributions of fibrin to fibrinolysis. TAFI is activated (TAFIa) by thrombomodulin-associated thrombin, which then cleaves lysine residues on the fibrin clot.[14] This results in a deceleration in plasmin generation, impairment in fibrinolysis and clot stabilization.

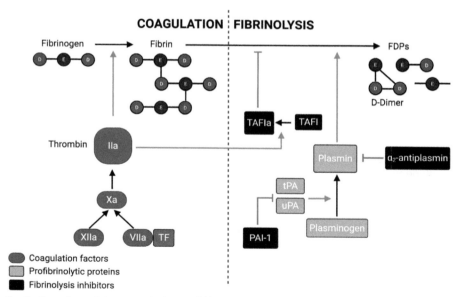

Fig. 2. Overview of the coagulation and fibrinolytic pathways. The formation of a fibrin clot is the end-point of the coagulation cascade. Subsequent degradation of the fibrin network into FDPs (eg, D-dimer) is mediated by the fibrinolytic system. Balance between these two pathways is essential in hemostasis, while abnormalities in these pathways may lead to bleeding and/or thrombosis. PAI-1, plasminogen activator inhibitor type 1; TAFI, thrombin activated fibrinolysis inhibitor; TF, tissue factor; tPA, tissue plasminogen activator; uPA, urokinase plasminogen activator.

CLINICAL LABORATORY EVALUATION
Fibrinogen

Abnormalities in fibrinogen may be initially suspected with prolongation of common coagulation assays including prothrombin time (PT), activated partial thromboplastin time (aPTT), and thrombin time. However, significant fibrinogen abnormalities are required to affect these assays, so dedicated studies of fibrinogen function and/or concentration are warranted when a fibrinogen disorder is suspected.

The Clauss assay is most commonly used to measure fibrinogen function. It requires mixing of dilute patient platelet-poor plasma with high concentrations of exogenous thrombin (to overcome any abnormalities in endogenous thrombin generation in the plasma), and measures the time to clot formation using a photo-optical system. Using a standard curve, the time is converted to a fibrinogen concentration and reported in grams per liter. Factors that reduce fibrin formation (eg, heparin, direct thrombin inhibitors) or factors that decrease light transmission (eg, hyperbilirubinemia, free hemoglobin, lipemia) can lead to inaccurate results.[15]

A PT-based assay (PT-Fg) can also be used to measure fibrinogen. In this assay, a PT assay is performed on patient platelet-poor plasma and compared to the PT from a series of plasma dilutions with known fibrinogen concentrations. Because of variability in reagents and instrument calibration, as well as the potential for overestimation of fibrinogen levels in qualitative disorders,[16] routine clinical use of this method is not recommended.[15]

Immunologic assays are available to measure fibrinogen concentration; this is most commonly performed via an enzyme-linked immunosorbent assay (ELISA). The clinical utility of an immunoassay is primarily in conjunction with the Clauss functional assay to identify discrepancies between fibrinogen concentration and activity, to differentiate between quantitative and qualitative fibrinogen disorders.[15,17]

Fibrinolysis

Multiple laboratory assays attempt to quantify fibrinolytic function, but assay interpretation and ultimate diagnosis of abnormal fibrinolysis is challenging as no true "gold standard" diagnostic test exists.[18] Here, we focus on the most widely used assays in clinical practice and conclude with a discussion of other tests that can be considered in specific scenarios.

Fibrin(ogen) degradation products and D-dimer

Fibrin(ogen) degradation product (FDP) is a broad term for the protein fragments generated during fibrin or fibrinogen degradation. D-dimer is a specific FDP that contains cross-linked D fragments of the fibrin(ogen) molecule. Measurement of D-dimer is used clinically as an indicator of endogenous activation of the patient's coagulation system and has been incorporated into diagnostic tools for venous thromboembolism (VTE), disseminated intravascular coagulation, and aortic aneurysm.[19] Over 30 different assays are commercially available to measure D-dimer, and there is significant variability in the units reported (fibrinogen equivalent units [FEU], D-dimer units [DDU]) and unit magnitude (μg/mL, μg/L).[20] Therefore, clinicians need to be aware of the units reported and the normal range from a given laboratory when using D-dimer thresholds from published literature for clinical decision-making.

Viscoelastic testing

Viscoelastic testing, including thromboelastography (TEG) and rotational thromboelastometry (ROTEM), provide dynamic measurements of clot formation, strength, and resistance to lysis. For both assays, whole blood is placed in a cup with a pin inserted and connected to a detection device (a torsion wire in TEG, an optical detector in ROTEM). As the pin moves relative to the cup (the cup moves in TEG, the pin moves in ROTEM), the detection device measures changes in resistance to that movement and creates tracings of those changes over time. Although attempts have been made to define reference ranges for viscoelastic testing,[21] values reflecting hyperfibrinolysis are not standardized or well defined; published examples are outlined in **Table 1**. These assays provide point-of-care flexibility but have significant limitations including operator dependence, lack of standardization, and frequent intersample inconsistency.[22,23]

Other laboratory assays to assess fibrinolysis

Assays quantifying individual components of the fibrinolytic pathway are useful in specific clinical scenarios, particularly in diagnosing congenital disorders. These include assays to quantify the concentration and function of PAI-1, t-PA, u-PA, TAFI, and α_2-AP.

Another class of assays measure functional characteristics. These assays rely on changes in the absorbance of plasma (turbidity) over time after initiation of coagulation.[24,25] The euglobulin clot lysis time (ECLT) developed in the 1950s is one of the original assays for global fibrinolysis assessment. A "euglobulin fraction" is created from patient platelet-poor plasma by removing fibrinolysis inhibitors (PAI-1, α_2-AP), while leaving profibrinolytic factors (fibrin[ogen], plasminogen, tPA), so that fibrinolytic activity can be measured.[18] Because this assay is complex and requires multiple processing steps, the ECLT has been largely replaced in clinical practice by TEG and ROTEM. Other plasma-based assays to assess fibrinolytic capacity use tissue factor or thrombin to trigger fibrin formation and t-PA to stimulate clot lysis and measure clot formation and lysis as an increase and subsequent decrease in turbidity.[26,27]

DISORDERS OF FIBRINOGEN
Congenital Disorders

Diagnosis and clinical manifestations

Congenital fibrinogen disorders (CFD) are rare and thought to represent about 8% of the rare bleeding disorders.[28] CFD occur due to mutations in *FGA, FGB,* or *FGB* that result in a qualitative and/or quantitative defect in fibrinogen.[29] These defects can be diagnosed using the Clauss assay and an antigenic fibrinogen level (as described in section *Fibrinogen*). Traditionally, CFD were classified according to functional and antigenic fibrinogen levels (italicized in **Table 2**).[30] Recently, the Scientific Subcommittee of the International Society on Thrombosis and Haemostasis (ISTH) proposed a reclassification of CFD based on fibrinogen levels and clinical presentation.[17] **Table 2** shows the reclassification of CFD and its clinical description along with references for more detailed information.

The clinical presentations of patients with CFD are heterogeneous, ranging from asymptomatic to bleeding symptoms of varying severity (easy bruising, menorrhagia, epistaxis, postpartum hemorrhage, postsurgical bleed, gastrointestinal bleeding, and rarely, intracranial hemorrhage).[31–38] Patients with CFD can also present with thrombotic events, with both arterial and venous thrombosis reported in up to 20% of patients.[39,40] Several factors are thought to contribute to the pathophysiology of thrombosis in patients with CFD, which include the absence/decrease of antithrombin-like properties of fibrinogen γ' (see section *Background*) and production of clots with abnormal fibrin structure.

Owing to incomplete penetrance, it is not uncommon for individuals with CFD to be diagnosed incidentally during routine coagulation assay testing or to present for

Table 1
Published measures of fibrinolysis using viscoelastic testing

Measurement	Abbreviation	Patient Population	Threshold to Define Accelerated Fibrinolysis	Reference
ROTEM®				
Maximum lysis	ML	Postpartum hemorrhage, trauma	>15%	[81,100]
Clot lysis at 30 min	LI30	Trauma	≤71%	[101]
Maximum clot firmness	MCF-EXTEM		≤18 mm	
Change in maximum clot firmness with addition of fibrinolysis inhibitor	ΔMCF-APTEM		>7%	
Total clot breakdown	X	Trauma	Within 30 min: fulminant hyperfibrinolysis Between 30 and 60 min: intermediate hyperfibrinolysis	[102]
TEG®				
Clot lysis at 30 min after maximum clot strength	LY30	X Trauma	>7.5% ≥3%	[103] [104]
Estimated percent lysis	EPL	Trauma	≥15%	[105]

Abbreviations: APTEM, assay on ROTEM that initiates clotting via extrinsic pathway with addition of aprotinin; EXTEM, assay on ROTEM that initiates clotting via extrinsic pathway with tissue factor; ROTEM, rotational thromboelastometry.

evaluation because of a positive family history.[31] Even so, individuals with CFD who are asymptomatic at the time of diagnosis, especially when diagnosed at a young age, may be at increased risk of future bleeding and/or thrombosis based on the type of CFD.

Women with CFD are also at increased risk of obstetric complications.[41] A systematic review of 188 pregnancies in 70 women with CFD between 1985 and 2018 found that 43% of pregnancies resulted in miscarriages, with the majority (76%) occurring during the first trimester.[41] Compared to the general population, these women also had higher rates of placental abruption (8% vs 0.5%) and postpartum hemorrhage (19.4% vs 2%–3%).[41]

Approach to management
Acute bleeding event. Owing to the rarity of CFD, recommendations for management are largely derived from expert opinion, and are dependent on the patient's clinical presentation and family history (**Table 3**).[42–44] Patients presenting with a major bleeding event, regardless of the type of CFD, should receive replacement therapy with fibrinogen derived from human plasma in the form of fresh-frozen plasma (FFP), cryoprecipitate, or virally inactivated fibrinogen concentrates.[42,43] Expert consensus recommends a target peak fibrinogen level of greater than 150 mg/dL

Table 2
ISTH classification of congenital fibrinogen disorders

Types and Subtypes	Clinical Presentation and Description	Reference
1. Afibrinogenemia (*quantitative*)	Complete absence of fibrinogen • Bleeding can occur in all tissues, including umbilical stump and muscles • Can uniquely present with spontaneous splenic rupture, poor wound healing, and painful bone cysts • Can present with thrombosis in large arterial and venous vessels	45,106–108
1A. Afibrinogenemia	Afibrinogenemic patients either with a bleeding phenotype or asymptomatic individuals	37
1B. Afibrinogenemia with a thrombotic phenotype	Afibrinogenemic patients with a thrombotic phenotype	36
2. Hypofibrinogenemia (*quantitative*)	Proportional decrease of functional and antigenic fibrinogen levels • Less symptomatic but can have major bleeding with severe hypofibrinogenemia (ie, fibrinogen levels <0.5 g/L) • Less thrombotic events than in afibrinogenemia	38,45
2A. Severe hypofibrinogenemia	Functional fibrinogen level <0.5 g/L	
2B. Moderate hypofibrinogenemia	Functional fibrinogen level between 0.5 and 0.9 g/L	
2C. Mild hypofibrinogenemia	Functional fibrinogen level between 1 g/L and lower limit of normal value	
2D. Hypofibrinogenemia with fibrinogen storage disease	Familial hypofibrinogenemia with histologically proven accumulation of fibrin in hepatocytes	109,110
3. Dysfibrinogenemia (*qualitative*)	Decreased functional and normal antigenic fibrinogen levels • Typically mild mucocutaneous bleed, associated with surgery, trauma or delivery	45
3A. Dysfibrinogenemia	Dysfibrinogenemic patients either with bleeding phenotype or with thrombotic phenotype not fulfilling criteria for dysfibrinogenemia 3B or asymptomatic individuals	31
3B. Thrombotic-related dysfibrinogenemia	Dysfibrinogenemic patient carriers of a thrombotic fibrinogen mutation[a] or suffering from thrombotic events with a first-degree familial thrombotic history (relatives with the same genotype) without any other thrombophilia	33,35
4. Hypodysfibrinogenemia (*qualitative*)	Discrepant decrease of functional and antigenic fibrinogen levels • Typically more symptomatic with severe bleeding and thrombosis compared with dysfibrinogenemia	32
4A. Severe hypodysfibrinogenemia	Antigenic fibrinogen level <0.5 g/L	
4B. Moderate hypodysfibrinogenemia	Antigenic fibrinogen level between 0.5 and 0.9 g/L	
4C. Mild hypodysfibrinogenemia	Antigenic fibrinogen level between 1 g/L and lower limit of normal value	

[a] Fibrinogen Dusart, Fibrinogen Caracas V, Fibrinogen Ijmuiden, Fibrinogen New York I, Fibrinogen Nijmegen, Fibrinogen Naples at homozygous state, Fibrinogen Melun.
Adapted from Casini et al; with permission.

Table 3
Summary of consensus recommendations for target fibrinogen levels depending on type of CFD and clinical situation[42–44,51,53]

Clinical Situation	Consensus Recommendation
Acute major bleed	• Cerebral bleeding: >150 mg/dL (peak) • Hemarthrosis: >100 mg/dL (peak) • Muscular bleeding without compartment syndrome: >50 mg/dL (peak) • For all other bleeds: >50 mg/dL (trough) until bleeding stops
Acute minor bleed	Consider antifibrinolytic agents[b]
Surgery, high bleeding risk[a]	• Preoperatively: >150 mg/dL (peak) for major procedure or >100 mg/dL (peak) for minor procedure • Postoperatively: >100 mg/dL (trough) until hemostasis is achieved • >50 mg/dL (trough) until wound healing is complete
Surgery, low bleeding risk[c]	Consider antifibrinolytic agents[b]
Routine prophylaxis	>50 mg/dL (trough)
Pregnancy	• >50–100 mg/dL (trough) once confirmed[d] • >150–200 mg/dL (trough) at the time of delivery

[a] Personal bleeding history or has afibrinogenemia.
[b] Antifibrinolytic agents include tranexamic acid and aminocaproic acid.
[c] If no personal bleeding history.
[d] If fibrinogen activity less than 50 mg/dL or with prior adverse pregnancy outcomes.

for cerebral bleeding, greater than 100 mg/dL for hemarthrosis, and greater than 50 mg/dL for muscular bleeding without compartment syndrome for patients with afibrinogenemia.[43,44] For all other bleeds, a target trough fibrinogen level of greater than 50 mg/dL is recommended until bleeding stops.[45]

As both FFP and cryoprecipitate require large volumes to ensure adequate replacement until hemostasis is achieved, fibrinogen concentrates may be a safer option, if available. The FORMA-02 and FORMA-04 studies demonstrated the efficacy and safety of fibrinogen concentrates for on-demand treatment of bleeding and as surgical prophylaxis in patients with congenital afibrinogenemia.[46,47] Currently in the United States, there are 2 concentrated forms of human fibrinogen, RiaSTAP (CSL Behring, Marburg, Germany) and Fibryga (Octapharma US, Inc., Hoboken, N.J.). Both are approved by the Food and Drug Administration for the treatment of bleeding in patients with afibrinogenemia and hypofibrinogenemia, but not dysfibrinogenemia.[48,49] The lack of approval for dysfibrinogenemia is due to the risk that fibrinogen concentrates could potentiate the thrombotic phenotype more commonly seen in dysfibrinogenemia. In a multicenter observational cohort study of 22 patients with CFD who were treated with RiaSTAP, thrombosis of the right cephalic vein was reported in a pregnant patient with dysfibrinogenemia (aged 35 years), who was receiving prophylaxis.[50] For patients with CFD presenting with mild bleeding events, the use of antifibrinolytic agents, such as tranexamic acid (TXA), may be sufficient for bleeding cessation.[42,43]

Surgery. For any surgical procedures, patients with a known history of prior bleeding or those with afibrinogenemia (regardless of personal history of bleeding) should receive prophylactic therapy to achieve a preoperative peak fibrinogen level of greater than 150 mg/dL for major procedures and greater than 100 mg/dL for minor procedures.[42,43,45,51] Postoperatively, a target fibrinogen level of greater than 100 mg/dL is recommended until hemostasis is achieved and greater than 50 mg/dL until wound healing is complete.[51] For surgical procedures associated with low bleeding risk, persons with CFD without a bleeding history (other than those with afibrinogenemia) may be managed conservatively without prophylactic therapy or consider the use of antifibrinolytic agents postprocedure.[43]

Routine prophylaxis. Most persons with CFD do not require routine prophylaxis. Expert opinions recommend initiating secondary prophylaxis in patients with afibrinogenemia or hypofibrinogenemia with activity levels less than 10 mg/dL who suffered a first life-threatening bleed, to maintain a trough fibrinogen level of greater than 50 mg/dL.[43] For recurrent non–life-threatening bleeds, initiation of secondary prophylaxis could be considered.[42,43]

Pregnancy. Owing to the high rates of obstetric complications, it is recommended that women with fibrinogen activity less than 50 mg/dL or with prior adverse pregnancy outcomes receive prophylaxis with fibrinogen concentrate once pregnancy is confirmed with a target goal of greater than 50 to 100 mg/dL.[42,43,52] It is generally agreed that the target fibrinogen level should increase throughout the pregnancy, but there is no consensus on the optimal target level. For women with hypofibrinogenemia (fibrinogen levels >50 mg/dL) or dysfibrinogenemia, *and* no prior adverse pregnancy outcomes, a rationale for using prophylactic fibrinogen concentrates throughout pregnancy is unclear. Generally, in the absence of prior bleeding or clotting history, expectant management is recommended.[53] However, it is worth restating that the risk of bleeding, thrombosis, and/or adverse pregnancy outcomes can be unpredictable in patients with CFD, even in the absence of prior complications.[54]

As the pregnancy progresses, trough fibrinogen levels should be monitored at least monthly in afibrinogenemic women, and ultrasound for monitoring fetal and placenta development is recommended.[43] For all women with CFD, expert opinions suggest a target fibrinogen level of greater than 150 mg/dL at the time of delivery for vaginal delivery and greater than 200 mg/dL for cesarean sections, and maintained for at least 3 days postpartum.[42,43,53] The efficacy and safety of such a strategy was demonstrated in a single-center case series of 12 full-term pregnancies in 11 women with hypofibrinogenemia (mean prepregnancy fibrinogen level 72 mg/dL). All 11 women received fibrinogen concentrates during labor and delivery, and reported no obstetric complications peri and postpartum.[55]

In addition, depending on the patient's thrombotic history and other risk factors for VTE (eg, obesity, family history, cesarean section), postpartum thromboprophylaxis should be considered in patients with CFD.

Thrombotic events. Patients with afibrinogenemia can present with thrombosis, as these patients lack the protective antithrombin-like activity of fibrinogen γ'. As such, it is recommended that fibrinogen concentrates be started concomitantly with the introduction of anticoagulation therapy in these patients. For arterial thrombotic events that require antiplatelet agents, concomitant fibrinogen concentrates are typically not indicated in patients with afibrinogenemia but can be considered if bleeding occurs.[43] For patients with hypofibrinogenemia or dysfibrinogenemia who present with VTE, anticoagulation alone is typically sufficient.

In terms of choice of anticoagulation, the use of low-molecular-weight-heparin is favored over the use of vitamin K antagonist because of the difficulty in monitoring the International Normalized Ratio (INR) when the baseline PT is prolonged.[43] Data on the use of direct oral anticoagulants in CFD are sparse, although some experts are open to this possibility.[43,56,57] Duration of anticoagulation therapy should be similar to guidelines for the management of VTE in the general population.[58]

Regardless of the type of CFD, thromboprophylaxis with low-molecular-weight heparin should be considered in high-risk clinical situations, such as surgery, or when fibrinogen concentrate is given, taking into consideration the patient's personal and family history of bleeding and thrombosis.[33,45]

Acquired Disorders

Diagnosis and clinical manifestations

Acquired fibrinogen disorders (typically hypofibrinogenemia) can present due to a consumptive coagulopathy (eg, disseminated intravascular coagulopathy [DIC]) or trauma-induced coagulopathy (eg, hemodilution after blood loss with volume replacement).[59–61] Liver disease can also result in hypofibrinogenemia due to reduced liver synthetic function or dysfibrinogenemia. Other causes of acquired fibrinogen disorders include medications (eg, L-asparaginase), malignancy (eg, multiple myeloma), the use of plasma exchange using albumin as a replacement fluid, and autoimmune conditions resulting in antifibrinogen antibodies (eg, rheumatoid arthritis and systemic lupus erythematosus).[62–65] Similar to CFD, patients with acquired fibrinogen disorders can be asymptomatic or present with either bleeding and/or thrombotic events. The heterogeneity in clinical manifestation is dependent on the etiology of the acquired fibrinogen disorder and whether other coagulation factors (both procoagulant and anticoagulant) are affected.

Acquired fibrinogen disorders may be suspected with a prolonged PT and aPTT, and subsequently confirmed with an assay documenting a low fibrinogen level. However, since fibrinogen is an acute-phase protein, the fibrinogen level may be within the normal range in acquired fibrinogen disorders. The term "relative fibrinogen deficiency" may be a more accurate description for hypofibrinogenemia in clinical situations where a normal range fibrinogen level actually represents a clinically relevant acquired fibrinogen disorder.[66]

Approach to management

In acquired fibrinogen disorders, management typically depends on the etiology. For patients in DIC with hypofibrinogenemia, adequate treatment of the underlying cause usually leads to resolution of the acquired fibrinogen disorder. Routine prophylactic use of fibrinogen replacement therapy based on low fibrinogen levels alone is not recommended. However, if there is active bleeding or a need for an invasive procedure, fibrinogen replacement therapy can be given to maintain fibrinogen levels greater than 150 mg/dL.[60]

In patients with trauma-induced coagulopathy with major bleeding and hypofibrinogenemia, the guidelines recommend treatment with fibrinogen concentrate or cryoprecipitate to keep levels greater than 150 mg/dL, with repeated doses as needed.[67] The use of FFP for the treatment of hypofibrinogenemia is not recommended due to the unpredictable amount of fibrinogen in FFP.[67]

As the liver is the site of production of the majority of coagulation factors, patients with liver disease typically present with impaired hemostasis from multiple coagulation factor deficiencies, in addition to hypofibrinogenemia and/or dysfibrinogenemia. Depending on the hemostatic defect, various procoagulant therapies can be used, including FFP, cryoprecipitate, platelets, recombinant factor VIIa, and prothrombin complex concentrates. The clinical rationale for each procoagulant is outside the scope of this review. In the setting of an acquired fibrinogen disorder from liver disease, routine correction of fibrinogen is not typically recommended.[68] However, in the presence of active bleeding or an invasive procedure, cryoprecipitate (favored over FFP to avoid the large volume load and adverse effect on portal pressure) is recommended to maintain a fibrinogen level greater than 100 mg/dL.[68]

DISORDERS OF ENHANCED FIBRINOLYSIS OR CLOT INSTABILITY
Diagnosis and Clinical Manifestations

Patients with enhanced fibrinolysis characteristically present with "delayed bleeding," meaning initial hemostasis is obtained after trauma or an invasive procedure (surgery, dental extraction), but bleeding develops hours later due to enhanced dissolution of the fibrin clot. Patients may also present with bleeding at sites with inherent increased fibrinolytic activity including the uterus (heavy menstrual bleeding), nares (epistaxis), and genitourinary tract (hematuria). Diagnosis is challenging and may be frequently missed, as standard laboratory measurements of hemostasis appear normal and dedicated testing (as outlined in Tracey A. Cheves and colleagues' article, "Laboratory Methods in the Assessment of Hereditary Hemostatic Disorders," in this issue) is required.

Congenital disorders

Congenital disorders due to an inherited absence or dysfunction of components of the fibrinolytic pathway can result in enhanced fibrinolysis (see **Fig. 2**). An overview of the diagnosis and clinical manifestations of these rare disorders is presented in **Table 4** along with references that provide more detailed information.

α_2-AP deficiencies are autosomal recessive and can be quantitative (type I) or qualitative (type II), permitting unregulated plasmin activity.[69,70] Patients with homozygous deficiency have severe bleeding phenotypes postprocedure or trauma, heavy menstrual bleeding, and intramedullary hematomas. Individuals with heterozygous deficiency are predominantly asymptomatic, although cases of bleeding complications have been reported with invasive procedures or trauma.[71] Testing for abnormalities requires both determination of antigen concentration to identify type I deficiencies and functional assays that measure the inhibitory activity of plasmin to identify type II abnormalities; activity levels less than 60% predict accelerated fibrinolysis with clinical bleeding in patients with acquired deficiencies.[72]

Similarly, PAI-1 deficiency is autosomal recessive and can be quantitative or qualitative, leading to excess fibrinolysis because of lack of inhibition of tPA and uPA. In addition to bleeding postprocedures, heavy menstrual bleeding, and postpartum hemorrhage, PAI-1 deficiency is associated with a significant risk of miscarriage and preterm birth.[71] Diagnosis requires measurement of PAI-1 antigen and activity, but both assays have important limitations.[71,73] PAI-1 antigen exhibits diurnal variation and therefore should be drawn in the morning.[74] PAI-1 activity assays are calibrated to detect increased rather than decreased activity and therefore cannot reliably identify pathologically low activity[75]; low PAI-1 activity levels (<1.0 IU/mL) have been reported in 10% of healthy volunteers.[76] Measurement of increased tPA activity can be helpful to confirm PAI-1 deficiency, although normal tPA activity does not exclude the diagnosis.[71]

Quebec platelet disorder is a rare autosomal dominant condition that results in gain of function of uPA and thrombocytopenia. The severity of bleeding manifestations varies, with some patients developing spontaneous hemarthrosis in addition to other characteristic bleeding symptoms of enhanced fibrinolysis.[77] Standard coagulation testing and serum uPA assays may be normal because in some cases, uPA concentration is increased in platelet granules but not in serum. Therefore, diagnosis requires dedicated genetic testing for *PLAU* duplication mutations in patients with strong family history.[78]

Acquired disorders

Acquired disorders such as DIC and trauma can result in decreased clot stability and/or enhanced fibrinolytic activity and lead to severe bleeding phenotypes.

DIC can manifest with thrombosis, bleeding, or a combination of the two[79]; a bleeding-predominant phenotype due to accelerated fibrinolysis is characteristically seen in acute promyelocytic leukemia[80] and postpartum hemorrhage.[81,82] Trauma induces variable degrees of fibrinolysis, with increased fibrinolytic activity associated with worse clinical outcomes.[83] Iatrogenic interventions such as the extracorporeal circuit in cardiopulmonary bypass increase fibrinolysis and can result in bleeding,[84] while enhanced fibrinolysis is leveraged with the use of exogenous tPA for thrombolysis in pulmonary embolism, stroke, and other thrombotic disorders.

Approach to Management

In patients with congenital or acquired enhanced fibrinolysis or clot instability, management of the contributing disorder is essential and often most effective to resolve the abnormality. In congenital disorders or when an acquired cause cannot be resolved, management hinges on the use of antifibrinolytic agents, which can decrease bleeding, reduce the need for blood products, and improve clinical outcomes. The unique management of individual congenital disorders is presented in **Table 4**.

The two most widely used antifibrinolytic agents are TXA and ε-aminocaproic acid (EACA). Both TXA and EACA are synthetic lysine analogs that inhibit fibrinolysis by displacing plasminogen from fibrin at the lysine binding site of plasminogen. TXA and EACA can be given orally or via continuous intravenous infusion, but TXA can also be given as a single intravenous bolus or used topically.

Antifibrinolytic agents have shown significant benefit in multiple clinical scenarios in which accelerated fibrinolysis or decreased clot stability contributes to increased bleeding, including trauma[85] and postpartum hemorrhage.[86] Guidelines recommend early administration (within 3 hours) of TXA for all trauma patients regardless of laboratory measures of fibrinolysis.[67] In postpartum hemorrhage, TXA is recommended for all patients with refractory atonic bleeding or persistent trauma-related bleeding.[87] Although 1g TXA is used most commonly, lower dose TXA meets pharmacokinetic and pharmacodynamic metrics and may be effective for prophylaxis.[88] Empiric use of antifibrinolytics has also been recommended in specific surgical scenarios to decrease transfusion requirements including cardiac[89] and orthopedic surgery.[90] Dosing varies significantly in published trials and for each indication, with dominant examples outlined in **Table 5**.

Importantly, there are also published examples that challenge the broad efficacy of antifibrinolytics in improving outcomes in patients with excessive bleeding. For example, in a randomized trial of TXA (1g intravenous loading dose followed by 3g infusion over 24 hours) versus placebo in patients with acute gastrointestinal bleeding, TXA did not improve bleeding-related mortality.[91] As a result, widespread empirical use of antifibrinolytic agents in the absence of trial data is discouraged.

Most patients tolerate antifibrinolytic agents without complications. However, studies have raised concern about seizure risk with TXA in cardiac surgery,[92] potentially due to structural similarities with gamma-aminobutyric acid (GABA) and/or glycine neurotransmitters. It is unclear if seizure contributes to increased mortality, and the limited data available suggest no long-term neurologic sequelae in patients after a seizure event.[93] There are also concerns about the potential for antifibrinolytics to increase the risk of thrombosis. Clinical trials do not consistently demonstrate an increased incidence in VTE,[85,86,94] although the risk may be increased in some populations[95] and with specific dosing strategies.[91] This has been a particular concern for VTE risk in women with refractory heavy menstrual bleeding who are also receiving

Table 4
Congenital disorders of fibrinolysis

Disorder	Inheritance Pattern	Subtypes	Diagnostic Testing	Clinical Presentation	Management	Reference
α_2-AP deficiency	Autosomal recessive	• Type I: Quantitative • Type II: Qualitative	• Antigen and activity levels	• Heterozygous: Asymptomatic, rare bleeding with procedures/trauma • Homozygous: Severe bleeding, intramedullary hematomas	• Antifibrinolytic agents • Fresh-frozen plasma	69
PAI-1 deficiency	Autosomal recessive	• Quantitative • Qualitative	• Antigen and activity levels • Free tPA antigen	Mild-to-moderate bleeding, heavy menstrual bleeding, miscarriage, delayed bleeding after injury/surgery	Antifibrinolytic agents	75
uPA excess, QPD	Autosomal dominant		• Platelet count (low in 50%) • *PLAU* duplication mutation testing	Variable phenotypes within families but severe bleeding and spontaneous hematomas possible	Antifibrinolytic agents	77

Abbreviations: α_2-AP, α_2-antiplasmin; PAI-1, plasminogen activator inhibitor type 1; QPD, Quebec platelet disorder; tPA, tissue plasminogen activator; uPA, urokinase plasminogen activator.

Table 5
Dosing of antifibrinolytic agents in specific clinical scenarios

Indication	EACA	TXA
Trauma	X	1 g bolus within 8 h of injury followed by 1 g infusion over 8 h[85]
Postpartum hemorrhage	X	1 g bolus with second 1 g bolus if continued bleeding after 30 m or rebleeding within 24 h[86]
Cardiac surgery	100 mg/kg bolus to patient, 5 mg/kg to CPB prime, followed by continuous infusion of 30 mg/kg during surgery[93]	*High dose*: 30 mg/kg bolus to patient, 2 mg/kg to CPB prime, followed by continuous infusion of 16 mg/kg during surgery[93] *Low dose*: 10 mg/kg bolus to patient, 1–2 mg to CPB prime, followed by continuous infusion of 1 mg/kg during surgery[93]
Orthopedic surgery	*THA, TKA:* 5 g bolus if <50 kg, 10 g bolus if >50 kg[111,112]	*THA:* 10–30 mg/kg ± repeat bolus or infusion[94]; 1 g bolus[111] *TKA:* 1g bolus[112]
Heavy menstrual bleeding	X	1g PO four times daily on days 1–4[113]; 1.3 g PO 3 times daily for up to 5 d with adjustment for creatinine >/1.4 mg/dL[114]

Abbreviations: CPB, cardio-pulmonary bypass; EACA, ε-aminocaproic acid; PO, oral administration; THA, total hip arthroplasty; TKA, total knee arthroplasty; x, no trials or recommendations identified; TXA, tranexamic acid.

combined hormonal contraceptives, but the clinical experience continues to suggest that the combination is safe and effective in women without an inherited thrombophilia or history of thrombosis.[96,97]

Topical TXA can also be considered in certain clinical scenarios. A meta-analysis in primarily surgical patients suggests that topical TXA reduces bleeding and blood transfusions, but the analysis raised concern about potential thrombotic risks that could not be quantified.[98] Data on epistaxis are unclear, with some suggestion of benefit, but limited by a lack of recent robust randomized controlled trials since new techniques in nasal cauterization, packing, and others have been incorporated.[99]

SUMMARY

Congenital and acquired disorders in fibrinogen concentration and/or function can increase the risk of bleeding and/or thrombosis, reflecting the complex role of fibrin(ogen) in coagulation and the fibrinolytic system. Depending on the clinical situation, fibrinogen concentrates may be used to achieve hemostatic control in congenital and acquired fibrinogen disorders. Global fibrinolysis assays are increasingly being used in clinical practice, yet because of their significant limitations, disorders involving clot instability and enhanced fibrinolysis remain challenging to diagnose. Antifibrinolytics remain the mainstay of treatment for both congenital and acquired disorders of enhanced fibrinolysis.

CLINICS CARE POINTS

- Disorders in fibrinogen concentration and/or function can increase the risk of bleeding and/or thrombosis.

- Depending on the clinical situation, fibrinogen concentrates may be used to achieve hemostatic control in fibrinogen disorders.
- Disorders of fibrinolysis can be congenital or acquired secondary to various clinical situations including trauma, malignancy, or sepsis.
- Antifibrinolytics are a mainstay of treatment for disorders of enhanced fibrinolysis.

ACKNOWLEDGMENTS

Figures were created with the help of Biorender.com.

DISCLOSURE

A.S. Wolberg has received research funding from Bristol Myers Squibb, Takeda, and Stago. M.Y. Lim reports receiving honoraria from American Society of Hematology, and consulting fee from Sanofi Genzyme and Argenx. J.E. May declares no conflict of interests.

REFERENCES

1. Weisel JW, Litvinov RI. Fibrin Formation, Structure and Properties. Subcell Biochem 2017;82:405–56.
2. Bennett JS. Structure and function of the platelet integrin alphaIIbbeta3. J Clin Invest 2005;115(12):3363–9.
3. Pieters M, Wolberg AS. Fibrinogen and fibrin: An illustrated review. Res Pract Thromb Haemost 2019;3(2):161–72.
4. Byrnes JR, Wolberg AS. Newly-Recognized Roles of Factor XIII in Thrombosis. Semin Thromb Hemost 2016;42(4):445–54.
5. Macrae FL, Domingues MM, Casini A, et al. The (Patho)physiology of Fibrinogen gamma'. Semin Thromb Hemost 2016;42(4):344–55.
6. de Bosch NB, Mosesson MW, Ruiz-Saez A, et al. Inhibition of thrombin generation in plasma by fibrin formation (Antithrombin I). Thromb Haemost 2002;88(2):253–8.
7. Fredenburgh JC, Stafford AR, Leslie BA, et al. Bivalent binding to gammaA/gamma'-fibrin engages both exosites of thrombin and protects it from inhibition by the antithrombin-heparin complex. J Biol Chem 2008;283(5):2470–7.
8. Allan P, Uitte de Willige S, Abou-Saleh RH, et al. Evidence that fibrinogen gamma' directly interferes with protofibril growth: implications for fibrin structure and clot stiffness. J Thromb Haemost 2012;10(6):1072–80.
9. Cooper AV, Standeven KF, Ariens RA. Fibrinogen gamma-chain splice variant gamma' alters fibrin formation and structure. Blood. 2003;102(2):535–40.
10. Domingues MM, Macrae FL, Duval C, et al. Thrombin and fibrinogen gamma' impact clot structure by marked effects on intrafibrillar structure and protofibril packing. Blood. 2016;127(4):487–95.
11. Cesarman-Maus G, Hajjar KA. Molecular mechanisms of fibrinolysis. Br J Haematol 2005;129(3):307–21.
12. Hoylaerts M, Rijken DC, Lijnen HR, et al. Kinetics of the activation of plasminogen by human tissue plasminogen activator. Role of fibrin. J Biol Chem 1982;257(6):2912–9.
13. Simpson AJ, Booth NA, Moore NR, et al. Distribution of plasminogen activator inhibitor (PAI-1) in tissues. J Clin Pathol 1991;44(2):139–43.

14. Mosnier LO, Bouma BN. Regulation of fibrinolysis by thrombin activatable fibrinolysis inhibitor, an unstable carboxypeptidase B that unites the pathways of coagulation and fibrinolysis. Arterioscler Thromb Vasc Biol 2006;26(11): 2445–53.

15. Mackie IJ, Kitchen S, Machin SL, et al. Guidelines on fibrinogen assay. Br J Haemoatology. 2003;121:396–404.

16. Jennings I, Kitchen S, Menegatti M, et al. Potential misdiagnosis of dysfibrinogenaemia: Data from multicentre studies amongst UK NEQAS and PRO-RBDD project laboratories. Int J Lab Hematol 2017;39(6):653–62.

17. Casini A, Undas A, Palla R, et al. Fibrinogen SoFXa. Diagnosis and classification of congenital fibrinogen disorders: Communication from the SSC of the ISTH. J Thromb Haemost 2018;16(9):1887–90.

18. Ilich A, Bokarev I, Key N. Global assays of fibrinolysis. Int J Lab Hematol 2017; 39:441–7.

19. Johnson ED, Schell JC, Rodgers GM. The D-dimer assay. Am J Hematol 2019; 94(7):833–9.

20. Longstaff C, Adcock D, Olson JD, et al. Harmonisation of D-dimer - A call for action. Thromb Res 2016;137:219–20.

21. Lang T, Bauters A, Braun SL, et al. Multi-centre investigation on reference ranges for ROTEM thromboelastometry. Blood Coagul Fibrinolysis 2005;16(4): 301–10.

22. Chitlur M, Sorensen B, Rivard G, et al. Standardization of thromboelastography: a report from the TEG-ROTEM working group. Haemophilia 2011;17:532–7.

23. Quarterman C, Shaw M, Johnson I, et al. Intra- and inter-centre standardisation of thromboelastography (TEG). Anaesthesia 2014;69(8):883–90.

24. Goldenberg NA, Hathaway WE, Jacobson L, et al. A new global assay of coagulation and fibrinolysis. Thromb Res 2005;116(4):346–56.

25. He S, Bremme K, Blombäck M. A laboratory method for determination of overall haemostatic potential in plasma. I. Method design and preliminary results. Thromb Res 1999;96:145–56.

26. Gidley GN, Holle LA, Burthem J, et al. Abnormal plasma clot formation and fibrinolysis reveal bleeding tendency in patients with partial factor XI deficiency. Blood Adv 2018;2(10):1076–88.

27. Pieters M, Philippou H, Undas A, et al. An international study on the feasibility of a standardized combined plasma clot turbidity and lysis assay: communication from the SSC of the ISTH. J Thromb Haemost 2018;16(5):1007–12.

28. Peyvandi F, Menegatti M, Palla R. Rare bleeding disorders: worldwide efforts for classification, diagnosis, and management. Semin Thromb Hemost 2013;39(6): 579–84.

29. Paraboschi EM, Duga S, Asselta R. Fibrinogen as a Pleiotropic Protein Causing Human Diseases: The Mutational Burden of Aalpha, Bbeta, and gamma Chains. Int J Mol Sci 2017;18(12):2711.

30. Neerman-Arbez M, de Moerloose P, Casini A. Laboratory and Genetic Investigation of Mutations Accounting for Congenital Fibrinogen Disorders. Semin Thromb Hemost 2016;42(4):356–65.

31. Casini A, Blondon M, Lebreton A, et al. Natural history of patients with congenital dysfibrinogenemia. Blood. 2015;125(3):553–61.

32. Casini A, Brungs T, Lavenu-Bombled C, et al. Genetics, diagnosis and clinical features of congenital hypodysfibrinogenemia: a systematic literature review and report of a novel mutation. J Thromb Haemost 2017;15(5):876–88.

33. Casini A, Neerman-Arbez M, Ariens RA, et al. Dysfibrinogenemia: from molecular anomalies to clinical manifestations and management. J Thromb Haemost 2015;13(6):909–19.

34. Castaman G, Giacomelli SH, Biasoli C, et al. Risk of bleeding and thrombosis in inherited qualitative fibrinogen disorders. Eur J Haematol 2019;103(4):379–84.

35. Haverkate F, Samama M. Familial dysfibrinogenemia and thrombophilia. Report on a study of the SSC Subcommittee on Fibrinogen. Thromb Haemost 1995; 73(1):151–61.

36. Nagler M, Kremer Hovinga JA, Alberio L, et al. Thromboembolism in patients with congenital afibrinogenaemia. Long-term observational data and systematic review. Thromb Haemost 2016;116(4):722–32.

37. Peyvandi F, Haertel S, Knaub S, et al. Incidence of bleeding symptoms in 100 patients with inherited afibrinogenemia or hypofibrinogenemia. J Thromb Haemost 2006;4(7):1634–7.

38. Peyvandi F, Palla R, Menegatti M, et al. Coagulation factor activity and clinical bleeding severity in rare bleeding disorders: results from the European Network of Rare Bleeding Disorders. J Thromb Haemost 2012;10(4):615–21.

39. de Moerloose P, Casini A, Neerman-Arbez M. Congenital fibrinogen disorders: an update. Semin Thromb Hemost 2013;39(6):585–95.

40. Korte W, Poon MC, Iorio A, et al. Thrombosis in Inherited Fibrinogen Disorders. Transfus Med Hemother 2017;44(2):70–6.

41. Valiton V, Hugon-Rodin J, Fontana P, et al. Obstetrical and postpartum complications in women with hereditary fibrinogen disorders: A systematic literature review. Haemophilia 2019;25(5):747–54.

42. Mumford AD, Ackroyd S, Alikhan R, et al. Guideline for the diagnosis and management of the rare coagulation disorders: a United Kingdom Haemophilia Centre Doctors' Organization guideline on behalf of the British Committee for Standards in Haematology. Br J Haematol 2014;167(3):304–26.

43. Casini A, De Moerloose P. Management of congenital quantitative fibrinogen disorders: a Delphi consensus. Haemophilia 2016;22:898–905.

44. Casini A, Neerman-Arbez M, de Moerloose P. Heterogeneity of congenital afibrinogenemia, from epidemiology to clinical consequences and management. Blood Rev 2020;48:100793.

45. Casini A, de Moerloose P, Neerman-Arbez M. Clinical features and management of congenital fibrinogen deficiencies. Semin Thromb Hemost 2016;42(4): 366–74.

46. Djambas Khayat C, Lohade S, D'Souza F, et al. Efficacy and safety of fibrinogen concentrate for on-demand treatment of bleeding and surgical prophylaxis in paediatric patients with congenital fibrinogen deficiency. Haemophilia 2021; 27(2):283–92.

47. Lissitchkov T, Madan B, Djambas Khayat C, et al. Fibrinogen concentrate for treatment of bleeding and surgical prophylaxis in congenital fibrinogen deficiency patients. J Thromb Haemost 2020;18(4):815–24.

48. CSL Behring. RiaSTAP Prescribing Information. Available at: http://labeling. cslbehring.com/PI/US/RiaSTAP/EN/RiaSTAP-Prescribing-Information.pdf. Accessed November 14, 2020.

49. Octapharma. Fibryga Prescribing Information. Available at: https://www. fibrygausa.com/wp-content/uploads/2019/04/Fibryga-PI_July-2017-2.pdf. Accessed November 14, 2020.

50. Lasky J, Teitel J, Wang M, et al. Fibrinogen concentrate for bleeding in patients with congenital fibrinogen deficiency: Observational study of efficacy and safety for prophylaxis and treatment. Res Pract Thromb Haemost 2020;4(8):1313–23.

51. Casini A, de Moerloose P. Fibrinogen concentrates in hereditary fibrinogen disorders: Past, present and future. Haemophilia 2020;26(1):25–32.

52. Saes JL, Laros-van Gorkom BAP, Coppens M, et al. Pregnancy outcome in afibrinogenemia: Are we giving enough fibrinogen concentrate? A case series. Res Pract Thromb Haemost 2020;4(2):343–6.

53. Management of Inherited Bleeding Disorders in Pregnancy: Green-top Guideline No. 71 (joint with UKHCDO). BJOG 2017;124(8):e193–263.

54. Peterson W, Liederman Z, Baker J, et al. Hemorrhagic, thrombotic and obstetric complications of congenital dysfibrinogenemia in a previously asymptomatic woman. Thromb Res 2020;196:127–9.

55. Cai H, Liang M, Yang J, et al. Congenital hypofibrinogenemia in pregnancy: a report of 11 cases. Blood Coagul Fibrinolysis 2018;29(2):155–9.

56. Margaglione M, Vecchione G, Cappucci F, et al. Venous thrombosis in afibrinogenemia: a successful use of rivaroxaban. Haemophilia 2015;21(5):e431–3.

57. Schreiber K, Sciascia S, Cohen AT, et al. Secondary thromboprophylaxis with rivaroxaban in major inherited thrombophilias. XXV Congress on the International Society of Thrombosis and Haemostasis Toronto, Canada; 2015, PO578-WED (ISTH Abstract). June 24, 2015.

58. Ortel TL, Neumann I, Ageno W, et al. American Society of Hematology 2020 guidelines for management of venous thromboembolism: treatment of deep vein thrombosis and pulmonary embolism. Blood Adv 2020;4(19):4693–738.

59. Bolliger D, Gorlinger K, Tanaka KA. Pathophysiology and treatment of coagulopathy in massive hemorrhage and hemodilution. Anesthesiology. 2010;113(5):1205–19.

60. Levi M, Scully M. How I treat disseminated intravascular coagulation. Blood. 2018;131(8):845–54.

61. Schlimp CJ, Voelckel W, Inaba K, et al. Estimation of plasma fibrinogen levels based on hemoglobin, base excess and Injury Severity Score upon emergency room admission. Crit Care 2013;17(4):R137.

62. Arai S, Kamijo T, Takezawa Y, et al. Acquired dysfibrinogenemia: monoclonal lambda-type IgA binding to fibrinogen caused lower functional plasma fibrinogen level and abnormal clot formation. Int J Hematol 2020;112(1):96–104.

63. Dear A, Brennan SO, Sheat MJ, et al. Acquired dysfibrinogenemia caused by monoclonal production of immunoglobulin lambda light chain. Haematologica. 2007;92(11):e111–7.

64. Liao KP, Sparks JA, Hejblum BP, et al. Phenome-Wide Association Study of Autoantibodies to Citrullinated and Noncitrullinated Epitopes in Rheumatoid Arthritis. Arthritis Rheumatol 2017;69(4):742–9.

65. Truelove E, Fielding AK, Hunt BJ. The coagulopathy and thrombotic risk associated with L-asparaginase treatment in adults with acute lymphoblastic leukaemia. Leukemia 2013;27(3):553–9.

66. Elliott BM, Aledort LM. Restoring hemostasis: fibrinogen concentrate versus cryoprecipitate. Expert Rev Hematol 2013;6(3):277–86.

67. Spahn DR, Bouillon B, Cerny V, et al. The European guideline on management of major bleeding and coagulopathy following trauma: fifth edition. Crit Care 2019;23(1):98.

68. Shah NL, Intagliata NM, Northup PG, et al. Procoagulant therapeutics in liver disease: a critique and clinical rationale. Nat Rev Gastroenterol Hepatol 2014; 11(11):675–82.
69. Favier R, Aoki N, de Moerloose P. Congenital alpha(2)-plasmin inhibitor deficiencies: A review. Br J Haematol 2001;114(1):4–10.
70. Matrane W, Bencharef H, Oukkache B. Congenital Alpha-2 Antiplasmin Deficiency: a Literature Survey and Analysis of 123 Cases. Clin Lab 2020;66(12). https://doi.org/10.7754/Clin.Lab.2020.200207.
71. Saes JL, Schols SEM, Van Heerde WL, et al. Hemorrhagic disorders of fibrinolysis: a clinical review. J Thromb Haemost 2018;16(8):1498–509.
72. Okajima K, Kohno I, Soe G, et al. Direct evidence for ssytemic fibrinogenolysis in patients with acquired alpha 2-plasmin inhibitor deficiency. Am J Hematol 1994; 45(1):16–24.
73. Jain S, Acharya SS. Inherited disorders of the fibrinolytic pathway. Transfus Apher Sci 2019;58(5):572–7.
74. Angleton P, Chandler W, Schmer G. Diurnal variation of tissue-type plasminogen activator and its rapid inhibitor (PAI-1). Circulation 1989;79:101–6.
75. Mehta R, Shapiro A. Plasminogen activator inhibitor type I deficiency. Haemophilia 2008;14(6):1255–60.
76. Agren A, Wiman B, Stiller V, et al. Evaluation of low PAI-1 activity as a risk factor for hemorrhagic diathesis. J Thromb Haemost 2006;4(1):201–8.
77. Blavignac J, Bunimov N, Rivard GE, et al. Quebec platelet disorder: Update on pathogenesis, diagnosis, and treatment. Semin Thromb Hemost 2011;37: 713–20.
78. Kahr WH, Zheng S, Sheth P, et al. Platelets from patients with the Quebec platelet disorder contain and secrete abnormal amounts of urokinase-type plasminogen activator. Blood. 2001;98(2):257–65.
79. Wada H, Matsumoto T, Yamashita Y. Diagnosis and treatment of disseminated intravascular coagulation (DIC) according to four DIC guidelines. J Intensive Care 2014;2(1):15.
80. Arbuthnot C, Wilde JT. Haemostatic problems in acute promyelocytic leukaemia. Blood Rev 2006;20:289–97.
81. Roberts I, Shakur H, Fawole B, et al. Haematological and fibrinolytic status of Nigerian women with post-partum haemorrhage. BMC Pregnancy Childbirth 2018;18(1):143.
82. Thachil J, Toh C-H. Disseminated intravascular coagulation in obstetric disorders and its acute haematological management. Blood Rev 2009;23:167–76.
83. Raza I, Davenport R, Rourke C, et al. The incidence and magnitude of fibrinolytic activation in trauma patients. J Thromb Haemost 2012;11:307–14.
84. Hunt BJ, Parratt R, Segal H, et al. Activation of coagulation and fibrinolysis during cardiothoracic operations. Ann Thorac Surg 1998;65(3):712–8.
85. Shakur H, Roberts I, Bautista R, et al. Effects of tranexamic acid on death, vascular occlusive events, and blood transfusion in trauma patients with significant haemorrhage (CRASH-2): a randomised, placebo-controlled trial. The Lancet. 2010;376(9734):23–32.
86. Shakur H, Roberts I, Fawole B, et al. Effect of early tranexamic acid administration on mortality, hysterectomy, and other morbidities in women with post-partum haemorrhage (WOMAN): an international, randomised, double-blind, placebo-controlled trial. The Lancet. 2017;389(10084):2105–16.
87. World Health Organization. WHO recommendations for the prevention and treatment of postpartum haemorrhage. 2012. Available at: https://www.who.int/

reproductivehealth/publications/maternal_perinatal_health/9789241548502/en/. Accessed August 1, 2020.

88. Ahmadzia H, Luban N, Shuhui L, et al. Optimal use of intravenous tranexamic acid for hemorrhage prevention in pregnant women. Am J Obstet Gynecol 2020;225(1):85.e1-11.

89. Society of Thoracic Surgeons Blood Conservation Guideline Task Force, Society of Cardiovascular Anesthesiologists, Special Task Force on Blood Transfusion International Consortium for Evidence Based Perfusion. Update to the Society of Thoracic Surgeons and the Society of Cardiovascular Anesthesiologists Blood Conservation Clinical Practice Guidelines. Ann Thorac Surg 2011;91(3): 944–82.

90. Fillingham Y, Ramkumar D, Jevsevar D, et al. Tranexamic Acid in Total Joint Arthroplasty: The Endorsed Clinical Practice Guides of the American Association of Hip and Knee Surgeons, American Society of Regional Anesthesia and Pain Medicine, American Academy of Orthopaedic Surgeons, The Hip Society, and The Knee Society. J Arthroplasty 2018;33(10):3065–9.

91. HALT-IT Trial Collaborators. Effects of a high-dose 24-h infusion of tranexamic acid on death and thromboembolic events in patients with acute gastrointestinal bleeding (HALT-IT): an international randomised, double-blind, placebo-controlled trial. Lancet. 2020;395:1927–36.

92. Takagi H, Ando T, Umemoto T, group A-LioCEA. Seizures Associated With Tranexamic Acid for Cardiac Surgery: A Meta-Analysis of Randomized and Non-Randomized Studies. J Cardiovasc Surg (Torino) 2017;58(4):633–41.

93. Koster A, Faraoni D, Levy JH. Antifibrinolytic therapy for cardiac surgery: An update. Anesthesiology. 2015;123(1):214–21.

94. Sukeik M, Alshryda S, Haddad F, et al. Systematic review and meta-analysis of the use of tranexamic acid in total hip replacement. J Bone Joint Surg Br 2011; 93(1):39–46.

95. Johnston LR, Rodriguez CJ, Elster EA, et al. Evaluation of Military Use of Tranexamic Acid and Associated Thromboembolic Events. JAMA Surg 2018; 153(2):169.

96. Thorne J, James P, Reid R. Heavy menstrual bleeding: is tranexamic acid a safe adjunct to combined hormonal contraception? Contraception. 2018;98:1–3.

97. Chornenki NLJ, Um KJ, Mendoza PA, et al. Risk of venous and arterial thrombosis in non-surgical patients receiving T systemic tranexamic acid: A systematic review and meta-analysis. Thromb Res 2019;179:81–6.

98. Ker K, Beecher D, Roberts I. Topical application of tranexamic acid for the reduction of bleeding. Cochrane Database Syst Rev 2013;(7):CD010562.

99. Joseph J, Martinez-Deversa P, Bellorini J, et al. Tranexamic acid for patients with nasal haemorrhage (epistaxis). Cochrane Database Syst Rev 2018;12(12): CD004328.

100. Theusinger OM, Wanner GA, Emmert MY, et al. Hyperfibrinolysis diagnosed by rotational thromboelastometry (ROTEM®) is associated with higher mortality in patients with severe trauma. Anesth Analg 2011;113(5):1003–12.

101. Levrat A, Gros A, Rugeri L, et al. Evaluation of rotation thrombelastograhy for the diagnosis of hyperfibrinolysis in trauma patients. Br J Anesth 2008;100(6): 792–7.

102. Schöchl H, Frietsch T, Pavelka M, et al. Hyperfibrinolysis after major trauma: Differential diagnosis of lysis patterns and prognostic value of thrombelastometry. J Trauma 2009;67(1):125–31.

103. Thakur M, Ahmed AB. A review of thromboelastography. Int J Periop Ultrasound Appl Technol 2012;1(1):25–9.
104. Chapman MP, Moore EE, Ramos CR, et al. Fibrinolysis greater then 3% is the critical value for initiation of antifibrinolytic therapy. J Trauma Acute Care Surg 2013;75(6):961–7.
105. Kashuk JL, Moore EE, Sawyer M, et al. Primary fibrinolysis is integral in the pathogenesis of the acute coagulopathy of trauma. Ann Surg 2010;252(3):434–42.
106. Arcagok BC, Ozdemir N, Tekin A, et al. Spontaneous splenic rupture in a patient with congenital afibrinogenemia. Turk Pediatri Ars. 2014;49(3):247–9.
107. Rodriguez-Merchan EC. Surgical wound healing in bleeding disorders. Haemophilia 2012;18(4):487–90.
108. van Meegeren ME, de Rooy JW, Schreuder HW, et al. Bone cysts in patients with afibrinogenaemia: a literature review and two new cases. Haemophilia 2014; 20(2):244–8.
109. Brennan SO, Maghzal G, Shneider BL, et al. Novel fibrinogen gamma375 Arg->Trp mutation (fibrinogen aguadilla) causes hepatic endoplasmic reticulum storage and hypofibrinogenemia. Hepatology 2002;36(3):652–8.
110. Zen Y, Nishigami T. Rethinking fibrinogen storage disease of the liver: ground glass and globular inclusions do not represent a congenital metabolic disorder but acquired collective retention of proteins. Hum Pathol 2020;100:1–9.
111. Churchill JL, Puca KE, Meyer ES, et al. Comparison of ε-aminocaproic acid and tranexamic acid in reducing postoperative transfusions in total hip arthroplasty. J Arthroplasty 2016;31(12):2795–9.e1.
112. Churchill JL, Puca KE, Meyer E, et al. Comparing ε-Aminocaproic Acid and Tranexamic Acid in Reducing Postoperative Transfusions in Total Knee Arthroplasty. J Knee Surg 2017;30(5):460–6.
113. Preston J, Cameron I, Adams E, et al. Comparative study of tranexamic acid and norethisterone in the treatment of ovulatory menorrhagia. Br J Obstet Gynaecol 1995;102(5):401–6.
114. Ferring Pharmaceuticals Inc. Lysteda [package insert]. 2013.

Moving?

Make sure your subscription moves with you!

To notify us of your new address, find your **Clinics Account Number** (located on your mailing label above your name), and contact customer service at:

Email: journalscustomerservice-usa@elsevier.com

800-654-2452 (subscribers in the U.S. & Canada)
314-447-8871 (subscribers outside of the U.S. & Canada)

Fax number: 314-447-8029

Elsevier Health Sciences Division
Subscription Customer Service
3251 Riverport Lane
Maryland Heights, MO 63043

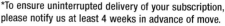

ELSEVIER